Managing Emergencies in the Outpatient Setting

Gregory M. Booth • Sarah Frattali
Editors

Managing Emergencies in the Outpatient Setting

Pearls for Primary Care

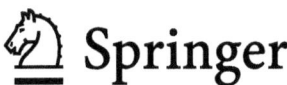

Editors
Gregory M. Booth
Baltimore, MD, USA

Sarah Frattali
Hampstead, MD, USA

ISBN 978-3-031-15269-6   ISBN 978-3-031-15270-2 (eBook)
https://doi.org/10.1007/978-3-031-15270-2

© The Editor(s) (if applicable) and The Author(s), under exclusive license to Springer Nature Switzerland AG 2022

This work is subject to copyright. All rights are solely and exclusively licensed by the Publisher, whether the whole or part of the material is concerned, specifically the rights of translation, reprinting, reuse of illustrations, recitation, broadcasting, reproduction on microfilms or in any other physical way, and transmission or information storage and retrieval, electronic adaptation, computer software, or by similar or dissimilar methodology now known or hereafter developed.

The use of general descriptive names, registered names, trademarks, service marks, etc. in this publication does not imply, even in the absence of a specific statement, that such names are exempt from the relevant protective laws and regulations and therefore free for general use.

The publisher, the authors, and the editors are safe to assume that the advice and information in this book are believed to be true and accurate at the date of publication. Neither the publisher nor the authors or the editors give a warranty, expressed or implied, with respect to the material contained herein or for any errors or omissions that may have been made. The publisher remains neutral with regard to jurisdictional claims in published maps and institutional affiliations.

This Springer imprint is published by the registered company Springer Nature Switzerland AG
The registered company address is: Gewerbestrasse 11, 6330 Cham, Switzerland

This book is dedicated to my family without whom this could not be possible.

Preface

This book is for providers in the field of primary care. Primary care clinics and urgent care centers are presented with challenging patients on a regular basis that cannot be discharged safely to home. Sometimes these patients have obvious presentations based on extreme pain, fevers, unstable vital signs, etc. However, occasionally the presentation is ambiguous or even difficult to discern. This book is meant to provide useful information in these cases where it is unclear when the patient needs to be managed in the emergency department or hospital. The decision to hospitalize often depends on local resources and availability of quick specialist input. Oftentimes, urgent referral for specialist input can obviate the need for an ED visit, though time constraints on clinicians make this impossible in many cases.

Doctor William Osler once said that medicine is the science of uncertainty and the art of probability. In this regard, this book gives basic information on the incidence and risk factors associated with the condition in question in order to ascertain its probability. Pertinent details about the history and physical examination will also be provided. Diagnostics in the forms of point-of-care testing (urinalysis, EKG) and also various laboratory and radiology studies will be discussed.

Several themes will be apparent upon review of this work. The immunosuppressed, especially diabetics and those on corticosteroids, are especially vulnerable and great care should be utilized when managing these patients. Additionally, it goes without saying that vital signs are vital. Anytime a fever, tachycardia, hypotension, or orthostasis is encountered, a red flag is raised. Finally, overreliance on diagnostics can lead to underdiagnosis and overdiagnosis. Studies should be ordered to help confirm the diagnosis and should be interpreted cautiously within the clinical presentation.

Although this book does not cover every possible situation, information on the most commonly encountered scenarios in primary care is discussed. Hopefully by reading and having access to this material, you will be able to quickly identify and manage emergencies in the outpatient setting.

Baltimore, MD, USA	Gregory M. Booth
Hampstead, MD, USA	Sarah Frattali

Acknowledgments

The editors would like to thank Emily Ball for help editing the manuscript and Olivia Welling for designing the illustrations.

Special thanks to Susan Tsu Thai for her careful reading of the manuscript and her constructive comments.

Legal Disclaimer

The following work is meant to aid in medical decision making and does not replace clinical judgment. The authors are not responsible for any uses of this material. This material does not address every potential situation that the clinician may encounter in practice. All clinical decision making must be weighed individually within the context of the patient's overall presentation.

Contents

Cardiovascular Disease. 1
Gregory M. Booth

Infectious Disease 33
Taisiya Tumarinson and Cynthia Rivera

Gastroenterology 75
Gregory M. Booth

Neurology 99
Gregory M. Booth

Nephrology 123
Gregory M. Booth

Urology 139
Gregory M. Booth

Obstetrics and Gynecology 153
Gregory M. Booth

Otolaryngology (Ear Nose and Throat) 165
Ioan A. Lina and Mark F. Williams

Pulmonology 185
Gregory M. Booth

Endocrinology 195
Gregory M. Booth

Hematology and Oncology 211
Gregory M. Booth

Ophthalmology 223
Gregory M. Booth and Susan Tsu Thai

Dermatology 239
Gregory M. Booth

Psychiatry 251
Gregory M. Booth

Index 263

Contributors

Gregory M. Booth Baltimore, MD, USA

Ioan A. Lina Department of Otolaryngology - Head and Neck Surgery, The Johns Hopkins University School of Medicine, Baltimore, MD, USA

Cynthia Rivera Department of Infectious Disease at FIU, Florida International University, Miami Beach, FL, USA

Susan Tsu Thai Baltimore, MD, USA

Taisiya Tumarinson Miami Beach, FL, USA

Mark F. Williams Department of Otolaryngology - Head and Neck Surgery, The Johns Hopkins University School of Medicine, Baltimore, MD, USA

Cardiovascular Disease

Gregory M. Booth

1 Introduction

Cardiovascular disease is one of the most commonly encountered groups of conditions encountered in primary care. Atherosclerotic disease in the form of coronary artery disease (CAD), peripheral vascular disease, and diseases of the aorta will be covered in separate areas of the chapter, with special attention to chest pain and CAD. Congestive heart failure and disorders of rate and rhythm will briefly be discussed. The thrombotic disorders of pulmonary embolism (PE) and deep vein thrombosis (DVT) will be discussed in detail. The commonly encountered syndrome of syncope will also be discussed in detail. Hypertensive urgency and emergency and its management will be addressed at the end of the chapter.

2 Coronary Artery Disease

Coronary artery disease is caused by obstruction of epicardial blood vessel(s) resulting in cardiac ischemia which can lead to tissue damage, a myocardial infarction (MI).

G. M. Booth (✉)
Baltimore, MD, USA
e-mail: Boothg444@yahoo.com

© The Author(s), under exclusive license to Springer Nature Switzerland AG 2022
G. M. Booth, S. Frattali (eds.), *Managing Emergencies in the Outpatient Setting*, https://doi.org/10.1007/978-3-031-15270-2_1

2.1 General Considerations

Ischemic heart disease is the number one killer in North America and Europe. Half a million people die from MI every year and an additional 700,000 thousand are diagnosed with unstable angina or non-ST elevation MI annually. A misdiagnosis of MI is still the number one cause of malpractice litigation in the USA.

Chest pain is a very common complaint and the causes are so varied that evaluation of risk becomes of paramount importance in managing patients in the outpatient setting. Some risk assessment tools are available such as the TIMI score and more recently the HEART score (see Table 1). Although the HEART score was validated for the emergency department setting, a brief review will give the outpatient clinician some points to consider when evaluating a patient with chest pain (see Table 1). Note that four or more points in the score results in admission to the hospital for a stress test. A highly suspicious (*H*)istory, (*E*)kg findings, (*A*)ge > 65, >3 (*R*)isk factors or history of atherosclerotic disease and (*T*)roponins >3 times normal are each given two points. Thus, the HEART score illustrates that historical items by themselves can identify patients requiring admission to the hospital for evaluation of chest pain, even those patients with a normal EKG or atypical chest pain.

At this point, it is instructive to note that an MI is defined by two out of three of the following: (1) Chest pain, (2) EKG changes in the ST segments, and (3) elevated cardiac enzymes. Therefore, a patient can have an MI in the presence of

Table 1 The HEART score is a numerical score for patients being evaluated for chest pain. A score >4 points is an indication for admission

*H*istory	Highly suspicious	2
	Moderately suspicious	1
	Slightly suspicious	0
ECG	Significant ST-deviation	2
	Non-specific repolarization disturbance/LBBB/PM	1
	Normal	0
Age	≥65 years	2
	45–65 years	1
	≤45 years	0
Risk factors	≥3 risk factors *or* history of atherosclerotic disease	2
	1 or 2 risk factors	1
	No risk factors known	0
Troponin	≥3× normal limit	2
	1–3× normal limit	1
	Lesser than or equal to normal limit	0
Total		

Abbreviations: *LBBB* left bundle branch block, *PM* pacemaker (Six, A.J. *Neth Heart J.* 2008)

a non-diagnostic EKG. Likewise, you can have an MI with non-classic presentations of chest pain, often seen in the elderly, diabetics, and women (see next section).

2.2 History

Differentiating cardiac from noncardiac etiologies of pain in the chest area is often difficult. Other considerations in this anatomic area are gastro-esophageal reflux and biliopancreatic causes, costochondritis, and pneumonia. Rare non-ischemic cardiac conditions like pericarditis (see below), aortic stenosis and pulmonary hypertension can also cause chest pain. Pulmonary embolism is a common entity and can mimic ischemic cardiac pain. Typical ischemic cardiac chest pain is intermittent (lasting 5–30 min), squeezing, and associated with exertion. Radiation to the arms, jaw, and teeth is common. Less specific symptoms such as abdominal pain, pain in one or both arms, shortness of breath, nausea, vomiting, diaphoresis, lightheadedness, dizziness, unusual fatigue, and overall sense of illness can be present. In contrast, atypical chest pain by definition is not associated exertion, but may have some of the aforementioned non-specific characteristics. Chest pain for seconds in the absence of other symptoms has an extremely low likelihood of being cardiac. Symptoms of heart failure may be associated with ischemic chest pain (see Sect. 4).

In known cardiac patients with angina, chest pain requires only continued outpatient monitoring if the same amount of exertion causes the pain and recovery time is the same (usually 5–30 min). However, chronic angina can become unstable and require emergent care. Unstable angina is defined as chest pain at rest, less exertion needed to cause chest pain, or markedly increased time necessary for recovery after exertion. A history of increasing need for nitroglycerin is also a symptom of instability, especially when used at rest. These patients should be considered for an admission for an ischemic evaluation. Unstable angina at rest is characterized by chest pain with typical features that occur at rest, lasts 20 min or more at a time, and occur frequently. These patients need immediate care.

The absence of chest pain can be seen with coronary artery disease (CAD), and the other less specific symptoms mentioned above (shortness of breath, arm pain, etc.) may be the presenting symptoms of CAD termed anginal equivalents. Liberal use of EKG should be used to rule out CAD when these symptoms are present, especially when in a pattern for typical cardiac chest pain. Sometimes the EKG (Fig. 1) itself will provide alarming indicators of a need for ED referral (see Wellens syndrome, Fig. 2) Sometimes patients will have had a previous evaluation for chest pain, and a stress test has some negative predictive value for 1 year and a cardiac catheterization for 5 years.

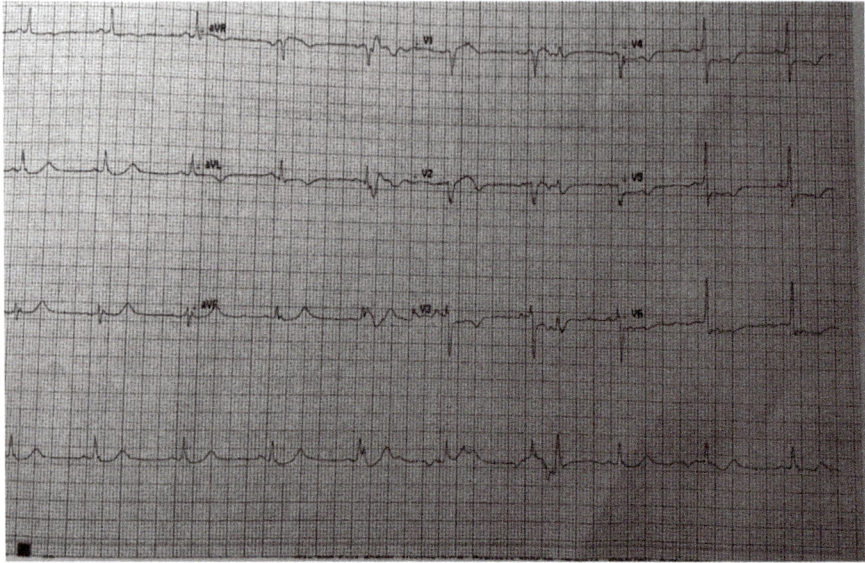

Fig. 1 EKG of a STEMI. Note the ST elevation in V1, V2, and AVR. Abnormal appearance in these leads is common but the presence of reciprocal depressions in V3–V6 made the EKG an emergent finding. The patient was a 73-year-old man with chest pain. Catheterization revealed an obstruction in his proximal left anterior descending artery (LAD)

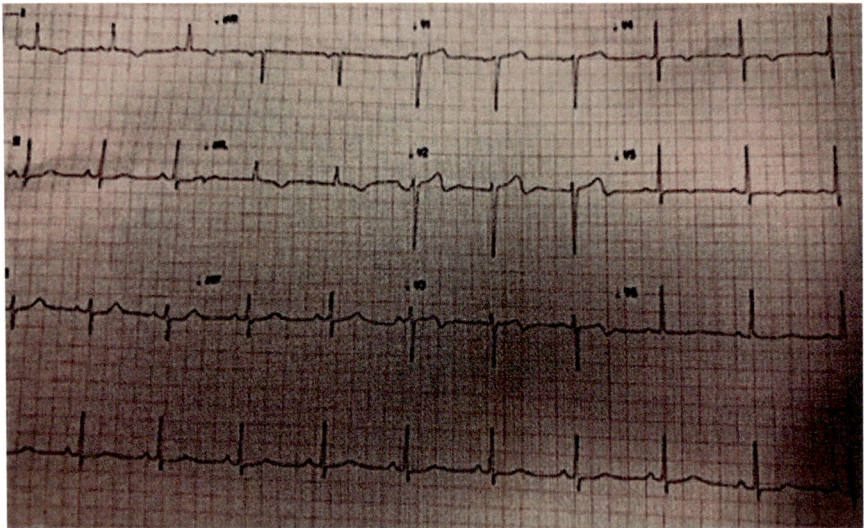

Fig. 2 EKG of Wellens syndrome. Note the biphasic T-waves in V1–V4 with normal R-wave progression. Wellens syndrome requires emergent treatment as it is a sign of severe coronary artery disease (CAD). The patient had minimal symptoms at the time, but catheterization revealed CAD with proximal left anterior descending (LAD) artery involvement. (Lee et al. *Am J Med*. 2021. Used with permission)

Cardiovascular Disease 5

2.3 The Exam

Tachycardia and bradycardia are often associated with cardiac ischemia. The fourth heart sound will usually be found with active ischemia. Signs of congestive heart failure may be seen (see below Sect. 4).

2.4 Diagnostics

If the patient is having active or recent chest pain and there are ST changes in two consecutive leads on the EKG (for example, see Fig. 1, an STEMI), then EMS should be activated for an acute ischemic event. The presence of T-wave inversions in the patient with active chest pain has a 20% chance of being an acute MI. The chance of MI with Q-waves on the EKG is even higher, up to 75%. Therefore, the presence of T-wave inversions or Q-waves in two consecutive leads should also be considered as ischemia in a patient with active chest pain. Of note, the Q-waves must be at least 0.04 s in duration (1 box on the tracing).

Key Points
- Patients with high-risk unstable angina (>20 min of rest pain occurring frequently) should prompt consideration for activating EMS.
- Patients over the age of 65 and with 3 or more risk factors or known cardiovascular disease should be managed with great care.
- A non-diagnostic EKG does not preclude serious heart disease.
- Inverted T-waves or Q-waves in two consecutive leads on the ECG should be treated as an MI in the right clinical context.
- Liberal use of EKG for possible anginal equivalents is necessary (especially in women, diabetics, and the elderly).

3 Pericarditis

Pericarditis is inflammation of the pericardium, the thin fibrous layer of connective tissue surrounding the heart.

3.1 General Considerations

Pericarditis is a rare condition accounting for 1 in every 1000 hospital admissions for chest pain and it is more common in men. The list of causes of pericarditis is long but can be divided into several main categories. A viral etiology is most common with coxsackie A and B and echo viruses predominating, but other viral causes such as influenza and the enteroviruses also occur. Bacterial (usually associated with pneumonia) and fungal pericarditis occur rarely. Pericarditis can also be seen with collagen vascular diseases such as lupus and rheumatoid arthritis. Post-MI pericarditis is an acute syndrome that occurs several weeks to months after MI and is called Dressler's syndrome. Cancer, especially lung, breast, and blood cancers can cause pericarditis, often in conjunction with a pericardial effusion. Pericarditis can cause tamponade, an emergent condition that arises when a pericardial effusion impairs diastolic filling of the heart resulting in acute heart failure. Bacterial and neoplastic pericarditis are often associated with tamponade.

3.2 History

Significant fevers may be reported, especially with bacterial and tuberculous pericarditis. The viral pericarditis commonly seen in young adults occurs about 1–2 weeks after a respiratory illness. Viral pericarditis is usually associated with low-grade fever, myalgias, and shortness of breath due to inability to take a deep breath from the severe pleuritic chest pain. The chest pain of pericarditis is ameliorated by leaning forward and worsens when lying flat. The pain can also be worsened by swallowing and may be present in the neck and shoulder blades.

3.3 Exam

Fever may be present. Heart sounds in general may be diminished and difficult to hear if there is an effusion, and a friction rub may be present. A friction rub is a scratchy, grating, high pitched sound that can change in quality and intensity and is often intermittent. The warning signs for tamponade are pulsus paradoxus, jugular venous distention, and lower extremity edema. Pulsus paradoxus is >12 mmHg drop in blood pressure on inspiration (seen with manual measurement). Pulsus paradoxus is 98% sensitive and 83% specific for tamponade. Other causes of pulsus paradoxus are massive pulmonary embolism, tension pneumothorax, and severe COPD. If these signs are seen within the clinical scenario of pericarditis, EMS should be activated.

3.4 Diagnostics

The EKG may be normal in pericarditis. In the acute phase, the EKG shows diffuse ST elevation with PR depressions. Later in the course, the T-waves will be diffusely flattened or inverted. Sometimes the QRS segments will be diminished if there is an effusion present (see Fig. 3). Rarely (5% of cases), electrical alternans can be present which is non-specific. Electrical alternans is a regular differential excursion of the QRS complexes representing the exaggerated "to and fro" movement of an

Cardiovascular Disease

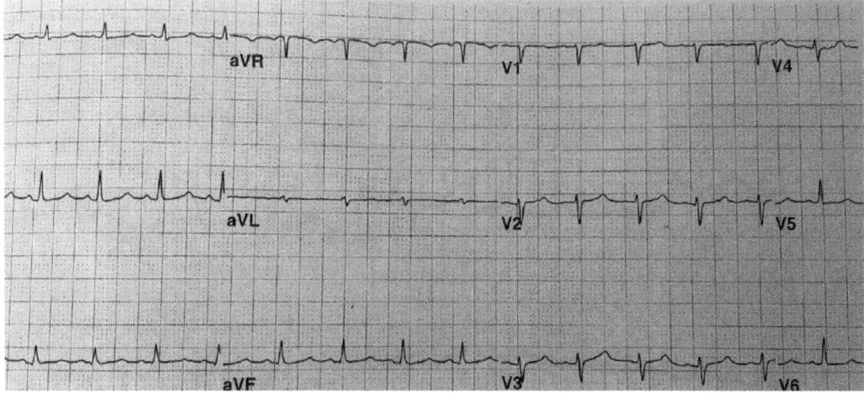

Fig. 3 EKG from a 51-year-old female with a pericardial effusion due to metastatic carcinoma of the breast. Note the low voltage in all leads except lead II. (From Surawicz and Knilans *Chou's Electrocardiography in Clinical Practice*. 2001. Used with permission)

enlarged heart. The chest radiograph may also reveal an enlarged heart and will show the classic "water bottle" shape.

Key Points
- The EKG can be normal in pericarditis.
- An emergent echo is often necessary to evaluate for the presence of a significant effusion (see Fig. 3). Furthermore, aspiration of pericardial fluid may be necessary for analysis to determine the cause of the effusion.
- In young patients with a history consistent with viral pericarditis and without pulsus paradoxus or signs of CHF, an outpatient approach may be followed.

4 Congestive Heart Failure

Congestive Heart failure (CHF) is characterized by fluid overload in the cardiovascular system causing dyspnea and edema.

4.1 General Considerations

Heart failure is a relatively common ailment with approximately a half a million new cases diagnosed every year. The etiology of CHF is varied, but the common pathway of the disease is a lack of effective pump action leading to fluid overload and/or lack of tissue perfusion. The cause of failure may be intrinsic to the heart muscle as in coronary artery disease or toxins such as alcohol. Other miscellaneous etiologies may affect the heart muscle such as infiltrative diseases like amyloidosis or sarcoidosis. Valvular dysfunction may lead to heart failure. Another potential cause is the complex interaction between heart rate and rhythm and the efficient, effective function of the cardiac pump (see Sect. 5). Some cases of CHF are idiopathic. In the outpatient setting, effective evaluation of the patient includes an assessment of the severity of the exacerbation and an investigation for an emergent etiology. In patients without a prior history of CHF, making the initial diagnosis is paramount for urgent or emergent management.

4.2 History

In addition to shortness of breath at rest or with exertion, dyspneic symptoms specific to CHF occur with the patient lying flat (orthopnea) or awakening at night short of breath (paroxysmal nocturnal dyspnea or PND). PND commonly occurs about a half an hour after falling asleep due to increased venous return while in a recumbent position, a similar mechanism to orthopnea. Other common complaints are less specific such as fatigue, presyncope, anorexia, and abdominal pain. Cough, insomnia, and depressed mood are also reported. A common precipitant of CHF exacerbations is dietary indiscretion, often with salt as the culprit. NSAIDs, alcohol, and noncompliance with medication are other common causes.

4.3 Exam

When tachycardia or bradycardia is present, strong consideration for a monitored setting should be entertained in CHF. The presence of murmurs should be sought. Jugular venous distention may be present. Signs of fluid overload are the most common with lung crackles or decreased breath sounds. However, the pulmonary exam may be normal with sub-acute onset of CHF. Ascites and lower extremity edema may be present.

4.4 Diagnostics

An EKG should be ordered to check for silent ischemia as this is a common cause for development or exacerbation of CHF. Arrhythmias (such as atrial fibrillation) may be involved (see Sect. 8). An emergent or urgent echocardiogram may be necessary to assess for valvular dysfunction as a precipitant of CHF. A chest radiograph may be ordered to assess for cardiomegaly or fluid overload but may be normal.

Key Points
- An EKG should always be obtained to check for silent ischemia.
- In cases of CHF exacerbations, patients with significant alterations in heart rate or a dysrhythmia should be considered for a monitored setting in the ED.

- CHF may have a normal pulmonary exam and lack of edema and a normal chest radiograph.

5 Arrhythmias

Arrhythmias are characterized by alterations of the natural rate or regularity of the function of the heart.

5.1 General Considerations

Arrhythmias will undoubtedly be covered in other material you study. Usually, malignant arrhythmias come to light in concert with other symptoms such as chest pain, shortness of breath, or syncope (see Sect. 17). These symptoms will play a role in deciding patient management. Ischemia often causes changes in heart rate, both bradycardia and tachycardia. In general, a ventricular rate >120 bpm should cause consideration for a monitored setting. The age and overall health of the patient plays a significant role in deciding management as higher rates can be tolerated in younger patients for longer periods of time. A common scenario is sinus tachycardia without cardiovascular compromise in a young patient with pneumonia. These clinical scenarios can often be managed as an outpatient. Bradycardia is often encountered in the outpatient setting and symptoms from bradycardia usually do not develop until the rate is between 35 and 40 beats/min.

6 Tachyarrhythmias

Tachyarrhythmias are arrhythmias characterized by an elevated heart rate and can be present in structurally normal or abnormal hearts. They usually come to attention with various symptoms.

6.1 History

The symptoms of these arrhythmias are palpitations, shortness of breath, or less specific symptoms such as fatigue. In severe cases, chest pain and syncope may be present.

7 Sinus Tachycardia

Sinus Tachycardia (ST) is a regular rhythm rate >100 arising from the sinus node.

7.1 General Considerations

Sinus tachycardia is generally secondary to a stimulus either abnormal (i.e., fever) or normal (exercise). Other innocuous causes of secondary ST are anxiety, caffeine, and nicotine. Another common etiology is alcohol withdrawal and its consumption should be evaluated in the history. Pathologic secondary causes include infections and cardiopulmonary causes such as chronic obstructive pulmonary disease (COPD), myocardial ischemia, and pulmonary embolism (PE). The association between PE and ST is very strong and ST is part of both the Wells Criteria for PE and PERC rule [see below under pulmonary embolism (Sect. 15)]. Once other more benign conditions such as anemia and thyrotoxicosis are ruled out, then the syndrome of inappropriate tachycardia should be evaluated with outpatient cardiac monitoring and prompt referral to cardiology.

7.2 Diagnostics

In the EKG, a p-wave will be before every QRS and the QRS will be narrow. The rate will generally be 150 bpm or less.

8 Atrial Fibrillation

Atrial fibrillation (AF) is characterized by a chaotic depolarization of the atria resulting in an irregularly irregular rhythm.

8.1 General Considerations

Atrial fibrillation (AF) is the most common sustained arrhythmia, found in 0.4–1.0% of the population. The prevalence increases with age and is found in approximately 10% of the population over the age of 80. Stroke syndromes are strongly associated with AF, and are found in 10–40% of new onset strokes depending on the age of the patient. AF is referred to as paroxysmal, recurrent, persistent, or permanent. Permanent AF is persistent AF which is no longer under evaluation for cardioversion or ablation. Sometimes AF is discovered in those with a structurally normal heart and without risk factors termed lone AF. If AF is encountered in the outpatient setting, the decision must be made to anticoagulate and this decision is based on a risk tool, the CHADS2-VASC score (see Table 2). In the absence of contraindications, a score of 2 generally indicates the need for anticoagulation. Anticoagulation can be accomplished with coumadin or novel oral anticoagulants (NOACs). Care

Table 2 CHADS2-VASc score. A score of 2 indicates need for anticoagulation in men. In women, a score of 2–3 indicates need for anticoagulation

Risk factors	Points	CHADS2-VASc score and annual stroke risk (%)
Congestive heart failure	1	1 = 1.3
Hypertension	1	2 = 2.2
Age > 65 years	1	3 = 3.2
Diabetes mellitus	1	4 = 4
Stroke/TIA/systemic embolism	2	5 = 6.7
Vascular disease	1	6 = 9.8
Age > 75 years	1	7 = 9.6
Sex (female)	1	8 = 10.8
		9 = 15.2

Abbreviations: *TIA* transient ischemic attack (Friberg et al. *Eur Heart J*. 2012)

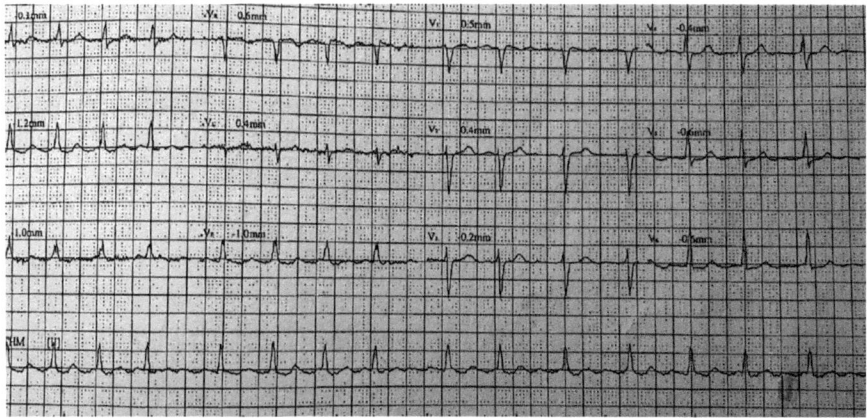

Fig. 4 Atrial fibrillation. Note the lack of P-waves and the irregularly irregular rhythm

should be taken that NOACs are properly dosed for age, weight, and kidney function. Many cases of AF are complex and need the attention of a cardiologist. Of note AF can be associated with PE, and careful attention should be made in this context.

8.2 Diagnostics

P-waves will be absent and the atrial depolarizations will be chaotic and fibrillatory in EKG (see Fig. 4). The rhythm will be irregularly irregular due to the variable conduction of the impulse from the atria. The QRS complex will be narrow.

9 Atrial Flutter

Atrial flutter is an arrhythmia caused by a macro-reentrant circuit in the right atrium and can also have an irregularly irregular rhythm.

9.1 General Consideration

Atrial flutter is the second most common tachyarrhythmia after atrial fibrillation (AF). Like AF, atrial flutter is also associated with cardiopulmonary disease similar to the conditions of atrial fibrillation (see above). Like AF, anticoagulation is generally considered according to the CHADS2-VASC rule.

9.2 Diagnostics

The EKG reveals "saw-toothed" p-waves and a variably conducted, narrow QRS complex (see Fig. 5). A case of flutter with 2:1 conduction is hard to differentiate from other tachyarrhythmias.

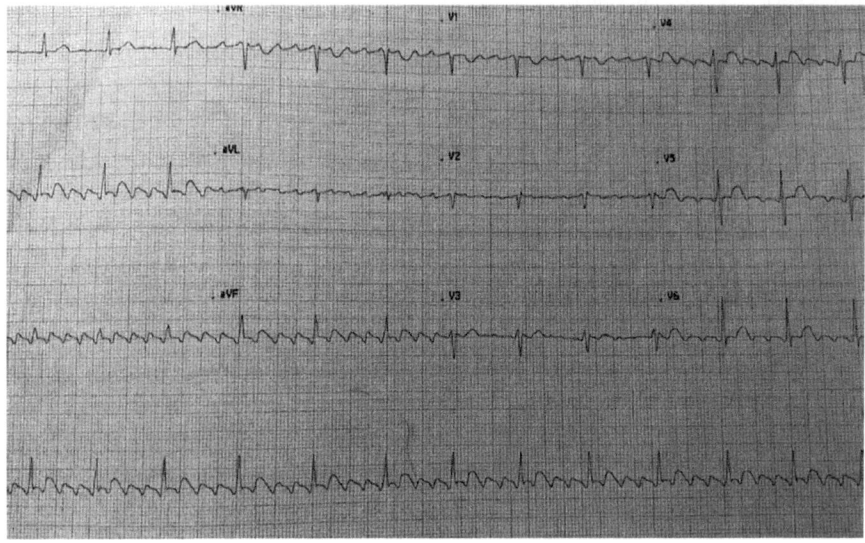

Fig. 5 Atrial flutter. Note the saw-toothed P-waves in the rhythm strip

10 Multifocal Atrial Tachycardia

Multifocal atrial tachycardia (MAT) is an arrhythmia characterized by p-waves of variable morphology and can be irregularly irregular.

10.1 General Considerations

Multifocal atrial tachycardia (MAT) is generally associated with chronic obstructive pulmonary disease (COPD) but can also be present with congestive heart failure (CHF). MAT is generally a disease of the older population and the therapy is treatment of the underlying cause. The rate does not generally exceed 130 beats/min.

10.2 Diagnostics

The EKG will reveal at least three different p-wave morphologies and will have a narrow QRS complex.

11 Atrioventricular Nodal Reentrant Tachycardia

Atrioventricular nodal reentrant tachycardia (AVNRT) is a tachycardia caused by a re-entrant circuit within the AV node.

11.1 General Considerations

Atrioventricular nodal reentrant tachycardia (AVNRT), commonly referred to as supraventricular tachycardia (SVT), is usually present in younger patients with a structurally normal heart and no cardiac risk factors. The symptoms are the same, however, with palpitations, shortness of breath being common. The condition can be associated with syncope or cardiac arrest when the arrhythmia terminates. The rate is generally between 150 and 250 beats/min.

11.2 Diagnostics

The EKG will reveal a narrow complex tachycardia. Sometimes the p-wave can be visible after the QRS complex.

12 Other Supraventricular Tachycardias

Other narrow complex tachycardias exist such as atrial tachycardia and sinus node reentry tachycardia usually seen in patients with structural heart disease. Atrioventricular reentry tachycardia (AVRT) is found in younger patients and Wolff-Parkinson White syndrome (WPW) [see Fig. 7 under syncope (Sect. 17)] can be considered a member of this class of tachycardias (most forms). WPW is characterized by pre-excitation which causes symptoms including syncope in 50–60% of patients. WPW can be complicated by AF which can cause extremely high ventricular rates which can deteriorate into ventricular fibrillation.

13 Ventricular Arrhythmias

13.1 General Considerations

Ventricular arrhythmias (VT) are not often seen in the outpatient setting but are still important to look for, nonetheless. The rate of VT can be quite low, and the patient can be asymptomatic. If your cut off for ED referral is 120 bpm, you should not be concerned about missing this entity. More comments about ventricular tachycardia will be made below concerning the rare syndromes of Long QT syndrome, arrhythmogenic right ventricular dysplasia, and Brugada's disease [see under syncope (Sect. 17)].

Key Points
- Supraventricular tachycardias are often seen with pulmonary embolism which is an emergency (see Sect. 15).
- Supraventricular tachycardias with a rate >120 need to be managed carefully and often will need emergent management.
- Atrial fibrillation with a CHADS2VASC score ≥ 2 needs anticoagulation if there are no contraindications. If there are any questions about management a cardiologist needs to be consulted.

14 Bradyarrhythmias

14.1 General Considerations

The sinus and AV nodes are usually supplied by branches of the right coronary artery and ischemia of this vessel can cause sinus bradycardia and various types of AV blocks. Sick sinus syndrome (tachy-brady syndrome) is sinus bradycardia mixed with episodes of atrial tachyarrhythmias usually atrial fibrillation. This is typically managed with a pacemaker. Pacemakers are usually set exactly at a rate of 60 (sometimes 50). Rates lower than this may indicate a malfunctioning pacer and these patients need to be promptly managed often with admission to the hospital if symptomatic. As mentioned previously, sinus bradycardia will be seen frequently and symptoms cannot usually be attributed until the rate is under 40. A symptomatic second or third-degree AV block usually requires pacemaker insertion.

14.2 Diagnostics

The EKG may find sinus bradycardia and second- or third-degree AV block. Sinus pauses of >3 s are always pathologic and shorter pauses often need immediate attention (see Sect. 17).

Key Points
- Bradycardias can be a sign of ischemia. If bradycardias are associated with cardiovascular symptoms, especially presyncope or syncope, management should occur in the ED.
- Malfunctioning pacers with less than baseline set rate (typical rates <60) need expedited evaluation.

15 Pulmonary Embolism

Pulmonary embolism (PE) is a thrombosis in the pulmonary vasculature.

15.1 General Considerations

Approximately a quarter to a half a million cases of PE occur every year. PE is common and will be encountered in the outpatient setting. Sometimes PE is massive (found in the main pulmonary arteries) and leads to cardiovascular collapse and death. Less serious thrombosis can form in the subsidiary arteries and can lead to a milder presentation which can be encountered in the office setting. PE has several non-specific symptoms and is one of the most challenging diagnoses in modern medicine, and a high level of susp`icion for this entity must be maintained. The Wells Criteria (Table 3) have been developed to estimate risk, with the most striking aspect of this tool is that shortness of breath without an alternate explanation receives three points out of a possible six which represents intermediate risk. While

Table 3 Wells Criteria for PE. Low risk 0–1, moderate risk 2–6, and high risk >6 (Wells et al. *Ann of Intern Med.* 2001). PERC rule (pulmonary embolism rule out criteria). When criteria are met there is <1% chance of PE in low-risk patients (Kline et al. *J Thromb Haemost*. 2008)

Wells Criteria	PERC rule	Risk factors for PE and DVT
Clinical signs of DVT (3 points)	Age < 50	Smoking
Unexplained shortness of breath (3 pts)	Pulse <100	Obesity
Heart rate >100 (1.5 pts)	SaO_2 > 94% on room air	Diabetes
Immobilization for 3 days (1.5 pts)	No hemoptysis	Oral contraceptives
Surgery within 4 weeks (1.5 pts)	No exogenous estrogen	Cancer
Previous PE or DVT (1.5 pts)	No previous DVT or PE	Pregnancy and post-partum
Hemoptysis (1 pt)	No surgery or trauma within prior 4 months	Trauma
Cancer with treatment within 6 months or palliative (1 pt)	No unilateral leg swelling	Immobility
		Post-surgical state
		Hypercoagulable states or previous PE or DVT

Abbreviations: *DVT* deep vein thrombosis, *PE* pulmonary embolism, SaO_2 saturation of oxygen

this must be contextualized with other risk factors, it is useful to keep in mind; i.e. acute onset of shortness of breath must be explained and serious causes ruled out. In patients under 50 years of age, the PERC (pulmonary embolism rule-out criteria) rule can be used to rule out PE in low-risk scenarios (see Table 3). Risk factors for venous thromboembolism are many. The most common and prominent risk factors are smoking, obesity, diabetes, oral contraceptives, cancer and pregnancy or the peri-partum state. Other risk factors are trauma and immobility, post-surgical state, and a hypercoagulable state (see Table 3).

15.2 History

The most common symptoms for PE are chest pain and dyspnea. Less specific symptoms include weakness and low-grade fevers. The chest pain associated with PE is often but not always pleuritic and can occur anywhere in the thorax, including the back, according to the area of infarction in the lung. Hemoptysis is also a classic symptom of pulmonary infarction. Syncope can occur especially in the elderly. PE resulting in syncope in the young usually implies a massive PE. The patient may relate the symptoms of a lower extremity deep vein thrombosis (DVT) such as leg edema, erythema, and pain. Sometimes, the chest pain and shortness of breath of PE resembles that of typical cardiac chest pain.

15.3 Exam

The patient may be hypotensive, and EMS should be activated if so. Fever may be present. The patient may be tachycardic and hypoxic. Even mild tachycardia (>100 beats/min) is concerning in this context, and a pulse oximetry of <93% or lower should be considered significant. The lungs may be underinflated in a massive PE and no sounds will be heard in the middle to lower lungs either unilaterally or bilaterally. The patient may have redness, swelling and pain in a single extremity, or rarely bilaterally, representing a DVT.

15.4 Diagnostics

Very little can be done in the outpatient setting to evaluate for PE. A normal D-dimer can be used to rule out PE in low-risk patients and can be useful especially if results are available the same day. An EKG can be used to evaluate for findings indicative of right heart strain. Right heart strain in the classic S1Q3T3 pattern is not commonly seen. Other findings are complete or incomplete right bundle branch block especially if new. S waves in lead 1 and AVL with Q-waves in lead III and AVF but not lead II is another EKG pattern associated with PE. Sometimes T-wave inversion in V1–3/4 are seen with PE (see Fig. 6).

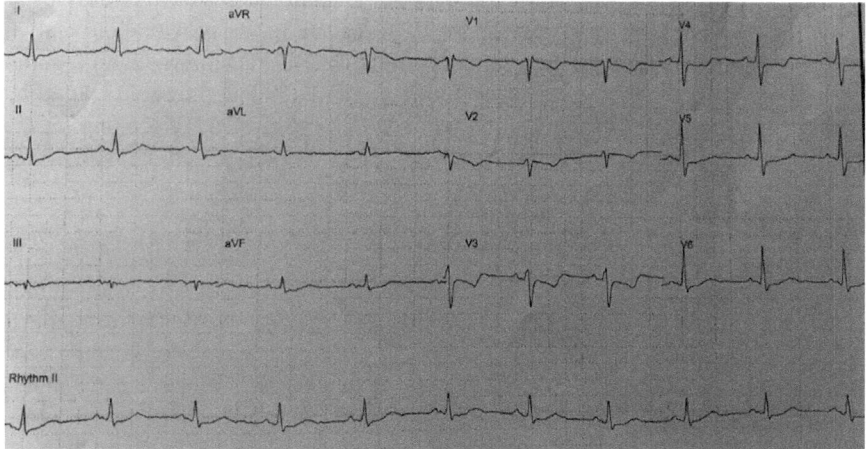

Fig. 6 A patient with PE. Note the inverted T-waves in V1–2 and abnormal T-waves in V3–V4

Key Points
- PE is a common but difficult to diagnose entity, and the clinician must be alert to risk factors, symptoms, signs, and diagnostic clues on the EKG as delineated above.
- The PERC rule can be used to rule out PE in low-risk patients under 50 years of age.
- Patients with a suspected PE should be sent to the ED. The patient should be examined for occult DVT.

16 Deep Vein Thrombosis

Deep Venous thrombosis (DVT) is a venous clot in the deep veins of the extremity.

16.1 General Considerations

Approximately 250,000 DVTs are diagnosed each year, and a high index of suspicion must be raised for this entity. The risk factors for DVT are the same for PE (see Table 3). Wells Criteria are also available for DVT (see Table 4). Proximal DVTs have a 50% risk of pulmonary embolization, especially upper extremity DVTs and up to 90% of patients with PE have a DVT. Calf vein thromboses have a much lower risk of pulmonary embolism, but 25% will propagate to the proximal circulation without anticoagulation. If there is a contraindication to anticoagulation, serial ultrasounds can be gotten to evaluate for propagation. A low threshold should be held for getting a Doppler ultrasound when DVT is suspected. Depending on the practice setting, many DVTs are handled in the outpatient setting with lower

Table 4 Wells Criteria for deep vein thrombosis (DVT). A score of 0 implies a low risk patient (Wells et al. *N Engl J Med.* 2003)

Wells Criteria for DVT (each worth 1 point)
Calf swelling >3 cm compared to the opposite leg
Entire leg swollen
Pitting edema (unilateral)
Localized tenderness along the deep venous system
Active cancer
Bedridden recently >3 days
Major surgery within 12 weeks
Paralysis or recent plaster immobilization of the lower extremity
Previously documented DVT
Alternative diagnosis as likely or more likely (−2 points)

extremity doppler ultrasound completed the same day and the initiation of novel oral anticoagulants (NOACs). A condition requiring emergent attention is phlegmasia cerulea dolens which occurs most often in the setting of cancer or hypercoagulable states.

16.2 History

DVTs can be asymptomatic. Most commonly pain and swelling in the extremity is reported. In the case of upper extremity DVT, a history of catheter placement is often reported.

16.3 Exam

The most common findings are pain and swelling. Swelling is defined by a 3 cm difference between the symptomatic and asymptomatic leg. Other findings are warmth, redness, dilated collateral veins, and a palpable cord. Homan sign is pain with flexion of the foot but is not a sensitive finding. Cyanosis can be seen with phlegmasia cerulea dolens.

16.4 Diagnostics

Doppler ultrasound is the test of choice and has a sensitivity of 95% and specificity of 98%.

Key Points
- Like PE, DVT is very common and can be asymptomatic.
- A 3 cm difference in leg circumference is the exam finding prompting further investigation.
- Lower extremity dopplers should be ordered liberally to detect DVT and have excellent sensitivity and specificity.

17 Syncope

Syncope is characterized by a temporary loss of blood flow to the brain resulting in loss of postural tone and consciousness.

17.1 General Considerations

Syncope is common and is responsible for 2% of ED visits. Syncope is not a disease per se but rather a syndrome with many causes. Cardiac causes of syncope will be our focus here; however, it is estimated that 6% of patients with syncope have had a transient ischemic attack (TIA) or stroke. Patients with a history or exam findings consistent with structural heart disease should always be referred to the ED as ventricular tachycardia must be ruled out in these cases. Syncope may be the initial complaint in 7% of patients who are 65 years and older with MI. Syncope may also be the initial symptom of pulmonary embolism (PE) in the elderly, and around 15% of cases of syncope in the elderly are associated with PE. As such, the elderly are more prone to potentially fatal causes of syncope and special care must be taken in their evaluation.

One of the most common causes of syncope is orthostatic syncope caused by volume depletion often complicated by medications such as antihypertensives. In younger patients, the cause of syncope is often vasovagal (also called neurogenic or neurocardiogenic syncope). Vasovagal syncope has many associations. Situational syncope is common, and micturition and defecation are common culprits. The postprandial state (within 1 hour), swallowing, coughing, sneezing, and laughing are also causes of vasovagal syncope. Carotid sinus syncope is rare (1% of identified causes) but should be considered in patients with syncopal symptoms caused by shaving, tight collars, and swimming. Other reported causes of syncope are prolonged standing, prolonged exertion, and tachycardia. Vasovagal syncope can be caused by pain or unpleasant sensory input (sight, sound, or smell). Another rare etiology of syncope is extensive arm exercise caused by subclavian steal syndrome. Subclavian steal syndrome should be considered in those with a >20 mmHg difference in arm blood pressures. In many patients, especially the young, the only evaluation a clinician needs is an EKG in the office which, if negative for any significant findings, will end their diagnostic evaluation. Bradycardia may be present [see under bradyarrhythmias (Sect. 14)] There are five other EKG findings to look for, especially in the younger patient: hypertrophic cardiomyopathy, Wolff-Parkinson White Syndrome (see Fig. 7), arrhythmogenic right

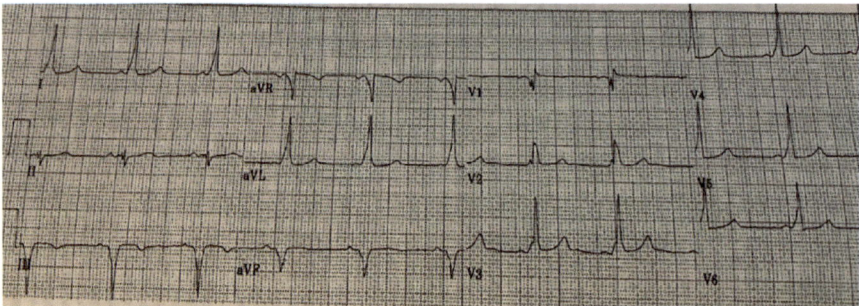

Fig. 7 EKG in a patient with Wolff-Parkinson's White syndrome. Note the short PR interval and slurred R-wave in Lead I. (Griffin, B.P. and Topol, E.J. Eds. *Manual of Cardiovascular Medicine* 2nd Ed 2004. Used with permission)

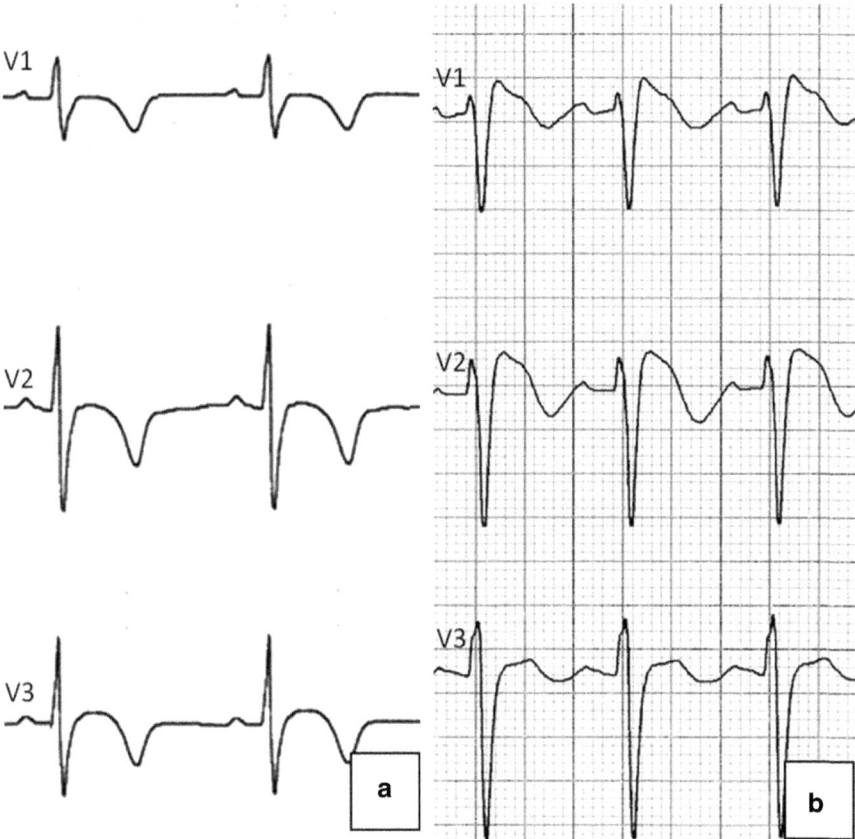

Fig. 8 (**a**) Arrhythmogenic right ventricular cardiomyopathy has inverted T-waves in lead V1–V3. (**b**) Brugada syndrome is associated with ST-elevation in V1 and V2. Both of these conditions are associated with syncope and sudden cardiac death. (Corrado, D. et al. *Circ Arrythm Electrophys.* 2016. Used with permission)

ventricular dysplasia (see Fig. 8a), Brugada syndrome (see Fig. 8b), and Long QT syndrome. These potentially fatal entities are thankfully rare and a careful glance at the EKG can rule them out. The most common among these entities is hypertrophic cardiomyopathy associated with a systolic ejection murmur and left ventricular hypertrophy (LVH). In up to 35–50% of cases, no cause for syncope can be found and the clinician must be satisfied in ruling out potentially fatal causes.

17.2 History

A family history of sudden cardiac death is an alarming historical finding. The patient will relay a feeling of "faintness" like I am going to "pass out" prior to the event. Cardiovascular symptoms should be evaluated such as chest pain and shortness of breath. One of the key historical distinctions to make is differentiating syncope from seizure (see Chap. 4 "Neurology"). The prodrome for seizure is an aura, often a sense of epigastric rising. Both syncope and seizure can cause rhythmic jerking movements; however, with seizure, the jerking movements generally last longer than 30 s. In syncope, the patients usually recover mental clarity much faster as seizures are complicated by confusion and lethargy after the event (post-ictal state). The prodrome for vasovagal syncope (the most common cause of syncope) is often nausea, a sense of warmth and diaphoresis which sometimes is confused with a seizure prodrome as these symptoms are common with hypoglycemia, a very common cause of seizure. A presence of headache before the event can be a symptom of a subarachnoid hemorrhage and when present, should prompt the clinician to obtain a stat head CT.

17.3 Exam

Bradycardia (discussed above) may be present and causative (a rate of <40 is generally necessary). Blood pressure should be taken in both arms to assess for a 20 mmHg difference in arms that may indicate subclavian steal syndrome. Orthostatic blood pressures should be evaluated with measurements lying and standing taken 30 s apart. A fall of 20 mmHg in systolic or 10 mmHg in diastolic defines orthostasis, but generally more significant drops in pressure are required for syncope. The presence of murmurs should be sought and a systolic ejection murmur can indicate either aortic stenosis or hypertrophic cardiomyopathy. Both are appropriate causes for referral to the ED in patients with syncope. Any signs of congestive heart failure (see above) should prompt ED referral as this indicates possible structural heart disease. A carotid bruit can indicate subclavian steal syndrome and should prompt ordering of a carotid ultrasound. A full neurologic exam should be performed and any focal findings should prompt an immediate head CT and MRI.

17.4 Diagnostics

A single resting EKG is diagnostic only 5% of the time but should be performed. Voltage criteria for left ventricular hypertrophy (LVH) should be assessed for hypertrophic cardiomyopathy (HOCM). Wolff-Parkinson's White syndrome is characterized by a short PR interval and a slurring of the R wave in the QRS complex most easily seen in lead 1 (see Fig. 7). An EKG consistent with arrhythmogenic right ventricular dysplasia (ARVD) reveals T-wave inversions in V1–V3 (see Fig. 8a). Brugada syndrome is characterized by ST elevation in V1 and V2 (see Fig. 8b). Long QT syndrome is characterized by a QT interval longer than 440 mm in men and 460 in women. Usually, the QT intervals are much longer in this congenital condition. Any signs of past or present ischemia (see above) such as new T-wave

Cardiovascular Disease 23

abnormalities, ST segment deviations, or Q-waves should prompt an ED referral. A fingerstick can be performed to evaluate glucose values in patients with symptoms of hypoglycemia.

Key Points
- Elderly patients (over the age of 65) without clear orthostasis or other precipitating cause should be referred to the ED to evaluate for PE and MI.
- New abnormalities on the cardiac or neurologic exams should prompt evaluation in the ED.
- Syncope and a sudden onset of headache require an urgent head CT.
- An EKG should be obtained in all patients and findings of hypertrophic cardiomyopathy (HOCM), Wolff-Parkinson White syndrome, Long QT or Brugada syndrome, or arrhythmogenic right ventricular dysplasia (ARVD) should be referred to the ED.
- Any new findings of ischemia on the EKG should also be referred to the ED.

18 Diseases of the Aorta

An aortic aneurysm is a pathologic dilatation of the aorta up to 1.5 times its normal caliber.

18.1 Abdominal Aortic Aneurysm (AAA)

18.1.1 General Considerations

AAA is common with a prevalence of 3% in those 50 and older. There is a strong male to female ratio (9:1). Risk increases in males after the age of 55 and females over the age of 70. The risk factors for AAA are those for other atherosclerotic diseases: hypertension, hyperlipidemia, diabetes, age, and especially tobacco use. In fact, the USPSTF has recommended that all males over the age of 65 who have smoked more than 100 cigarettes get a one-time screening abdominal ultrasound. Family history also has a role, as 28% of patients have a first-degree relative with AAA. Likewise, if a patient has a first-degree male relative with a AAA, the patient is 12 times more likely to develop AAA.

18.1.2 History

Most AAAs are asymptomatic and are found on imaging incidentally. Severe back pain or flank pain can indicate impending rupture. This pain can radiate into the legs, buttocks, or groin. The pain is often described as sudden in onset, constant, and non-positional.

18.1.3 Physical Exam

A palpable pulsatile mass may be felt on examination. Palpation should be gentle as tenderness can indicate impending rupture. Signs of vascular disease such as bruits and decreased pulses are sometimes found. Embolized fragments of atherosclerotic plaques are sometimes found in the lower extremities causing findings such as livedo reticularis and painful blue toes.

18.1.4 Diagnostics

Abdominal ultrasound is very accurate and can measure the size of the aorta to within 0.3 cm. It is also readily available. CT is also an excellent study and can reveal more detail about possible dissection or disease in branching vessels. Indications for surgery are a diameter >5.0 cm. (A growth rate of >0.5 cm/year indicates need for prioritized surgical evaluation).

Key Points
- Patients with risk factors should be evaluated for AAA as an outpatient.
- Patients with symptoms and a significant AAA can be sent to the ED for expedited evaluation of surgery.
- If a patient with risk factors is having unusual back pain, a same day study of either abdominal ultrasound or CT should be performed.

In the right clinical context, a tender pulsatile mass with abnormal vital signs and other typical symptoms would be indications for activation of EMS and deep palpation on exam should be avoided.

18.2 Thoracic Aortic Aneurysm

Thoracic aortic aneurysm is a dilatation of either the ascending or descending aorta.

18.2.1 General Considerations

Thoracic aortic aneurysm (TAA) is much less common than AAA. There is no gender predominance, but risk increases at the age of 65 in men and approximately 75 in women. There is a long list of diseases associated with TAA. Genetic diseases such as Marfan's, Ehlers Danlos, and Loyz-Dietz syndromes generally affect the ascending aorta. Atherosclerosis is the major cause for aneurysms of the descending thoracic aorta with its attendant risk factors (see Sect. 18.1.1). Various rheumatologic diseases (Takayasu arteritis, giant cell arteritis or temporal arteritis, and spondyloarthropathies) are also implicated as are infections such as syphilis and mycotic infections.

18.2.2 History

The history is often negative as most cases are asymptomatic. A gradual onset of chest pain can be reported. If the aortic root is affected causing aortic insufficiency (AI), the result could be symptoms of CHF. If there is compression of surrounding structures in the thorax, then dysphagia, dysarthria, cough, and wheezing may result.

18.2.3 Exam

There may be the diastolic murmur of AI, at the right lower sternal border and the signs of CHF. The constellation of changes to the pulses associated with AI may be present. Examination of the digits may reveal thromboembolic events. The signs of superior vena cava syndrome may begin (dilation of the neck veins). A bifid uvula is a sign of Loyz-Dietz syndrome.

18.2.4 Diagnostics

TAA is most commonly found incidentally on chest radiograph with widening of the mediastinum appreciated. Chest radiograph is 80–90% sensitive for TAA but CT is a more sensitive test. The cut off for surgery is less clear than in AAA. Many experts agree that around 5 cm (like AAA) is a reasonable cut off for consideration of surgical management.

Key Points
- Like abdominal aortic aneurysm (AAA), TAA is usually asymptomatic.
- Risk factors associated with suggestive symptoms or signs (see above) should prompt same day CT scan (either outpatient or in the ER).

A CT scan showing >5 cm or a widened mediastinum on chest radiograph should prompt consideration for ED referral if associated with symptoms.

18.3 Aortic Dissection

Aortic Dissection is a different entity than aneurysms and results from penetration of blood into the lining of the aortic muscle wall, usually in the ascending or descending thoracic aorta (the area under maximum pressure).

18.3.1 General Considerations

Aortic dissection is rare with about 2000 cases/year in the US. Hypertension is found in over 80% of cases. Age is also a risk factor. There are some similar associations to thoracic aortic aneurysms such as Marfan's and Ehlers Danlos syndrome as well as giant cell arteritis. Some unique associations exist such as Turner's Syndrome, bicuspid and unicuspid aortic valves, and coarctation of the aorta. Pregnancy and the peripartum state are important risk factors.

18.3.2 History

The chest pain associated with dissection is sudden and reaches extreme peak rapidly and lasts for hours. Chest pain is the most common presenting symptom seen 75–95% of the time. The pain is commonly described as a tearing or ripping sensation radiating to the back especially between the scapulae. However, the chest pain can be anterior with dissections in the ascending portion of the aorta. The pain is abrupt unlike that of a myocardial infarction (MI) which usually has a more gradual onset. Symptoms of congestive heart failure (CHF) can be present with severe aortic insufficiency (AI) (see below). Neurologic symptoms of CVA are present 3–6% of the time. Rarely, paraplegia can occur in descending thoracic dissections into spinal vessels.

18.3.3 Exam

Hypertension is commonly present. However, lower blood pressures and even hypotension may be seen in tamponade and hemopericardium from proximal dissection into cardiac vessels. Pseudo-hypotension can also occur when the dissection propagates into the subclavian artery and pressure should be evaluated in both arms. As with thoracic aneurysm, aortic insufficiency can occur due to interference with coaptation of the aortic valve leaflets.

18.3.4 Diagnostics

The EKG may rarely (1–2% of the time) show an acute MI with dissection into the coronary ostia as mentioned above with hemopericardium. Up to 80–90% of the time, aortic pathology will be seen on chest X-ray as in the case with thoracic aneurysm.

Key Points
- Aortic dissection is a rare condition most often seen in the older population with uncontrolled hypertension, but other risk factors exist such as those mentioned above.
- Dissection is associated with a variety of symptoms such as tearing, ripping chest pain, and occasionally CHF and CVA.

The chest radiograph has an 80–90% sensitivity for dissection as it does for thoracic aneurysm.

Cardiovascular Disease

19 Acute Limb Ischemia

Acute limb ischemia is a loss of blood flow to an extremity resulting in potential loss of viable tissue.

19.1 General Considerations

Acute limb ischemia is usually caused by atherosclerotic peripheral vascular disease (PVD) and has atherosclerotic risk factors such as diabetes, hyperlipidemia, hypertension, and especially tobacco use. The risk is highest in diabetics who smoke. Symptomatic ischemia affects approximately 2–3% of the older population. 70% of those symptomatic patients will remain stable or improve with exercise and lifestyle modifications. The other 30% will progress with approximately 5% requiring amputation in 5 years if not revascularized. The relationship between symptomatic PVD and cardiac disease is very strong as cardiac mortality is six times higher in this population. Patients with PVD should be referred to cardiology for evaluation.

19.2 History

Symptoms of claudication (symptomatic PVD) are pain, discomfort, or fatigue in the buttock, thigh, or calf muscles. Claudication is characterized by discomfort that always occurs with the same amount of activity and always relieved with rest. Claudication comes on gradually and symptoms are evident one level below the segment of severe stenosis with severity of symptoms roughly correlating to severity of stenosis. As such, buttock symptoms are due to aortic disease, thigh symptoms from iliac disease, and calf symptoms are due to superficial femoral artery stenosis which is the most common site of disease. The foot and toes are affected by disease in the tibial arteries. Rest pain not relieved by a dependent position of the leg, represents critical ischemia, and is an emergency. Rarely, acute limb ischemia is caused by thrombosis which is characterized by the sudden onset of the 5 P's: pain, paresthesias, poikilothermia (cold), pallor, and pulselessness.

19.3 Exam

The quality of all the pulses should be noted including the carotid, femoral, popliteal, dorsalis pedis, and posterior tibialis arteries. Auscultation for bruits should be performed in the carotid and femoral arteries. Other signs are loss of hair on the extremity, coolness of the extremity, pallor worsened with limb elevation, and dry skin with flaking. Dry gangrene is a blackening of the skin (eschar) or digit with a clear demarcation between dead and healthy tissue. Dry gangrene is a sign of critical disease but does not need to be seen in the ED if urgent vascular assessment can be obtained. Wet gangrene is dead tissue complicated by infection and is an emergency and should be referred to the ED. Wet gangrene is an infection characterized by swelling, discoloration of the tissue, and a foul odor.

Key Points
- Leg pain at rest typical of ischemia, which is not relieved by a dependent position, is an emergency and should be sent to the ED.
- Wet gangrene is a swollen, discolored infection with a foul smell and is an emergency.
- Limb thrombosis is associated with the 5 P's: pain, paresthesias, poikilothermia, pallor, and pulselessness.
- Dry gangrene is not an emergency and can be handled urgently within several days.

20 Hypertensive Urgencies and Emergencies

Hypertensive emergency is a dangerous elevation of the blood pressure resulting in end organ damage.

20.1 General Considerations

Hypertensive emergencies are always referred to the ED for management. Hypertensive emergencies are differentiated from hypertensive urgencies based on symptoms, signs, and diagnostics. End organ damage or dysfunction is usually caused by an abrupt increase in blood pressure. A risk factor is poorly controlled essential hypertension and an association of hypertensive emergencies has been found with renovascular hypertension in particular. Certain prescription drugs such as oral contraceptives, NSAIDs, tricyclic antidepressants, and monoamine oxidase inhibitors can be precipitating factors. Cold medicines with decongestants can also be culprits. Smoking is also a risk factor as are drugs of abuse such as cocaine and amphetamines. Rarer associations are collagen vascular disease and vasculitis. A hypertensive urgency is defined as a blood pressure of 180/110 or greater in the absence of symptoms or end organ damage and these patients also need to be managed with great care. Clonidine may be available in the office and can be used to reduce the blood pressure until an anti-hypertensive is started.

20.2 History

The cardiac complications of hypertensive emergencies are ischemia and congestive heart failure (CHF), resulting in chest pain and shortness of breath. Neurologic complications called hypertensive encephalopathy are characterized by headache, irritability, and altered mental status. Neurologic symptoms are insidious and occur over several days which help distinguish an acute stroke from hypertensive encephalopathy. Visual disturbances can occur such as double vision. Gastrointestinal symptoms can occur such as anorexia, nausea, and abdominal pain. Back pain is also concerning for dissection.

20.3 Exam

Blood pressure in both arms should be checked. A thorough neurologic exam should be performed looking for focal signs. The cardiac exam should show an S4 and signs of CHF may be present.

20.4 Diagnostics

The EKG may show signs of ischemia or a new strain pattern. The urinalysis can show blood and 2+ protein.

Key Points
- Patients with very elevated blood pressure associated with typical symptoms of hypertensive emergencies should be seen in the ED, especially when signs or diagnostics are present as well.
- In clear circumstances, symptomatic patients are managed in the ICU/CCU and activating EMS is appropriate.
- Elevations in the clinic of blood pressure to 180 systolic or 110 diastolic should have an EKG and urinalysis done to check for organ dysfunction and, if found, should be sent to the ED.

21 Rheumatic Fever

Rheumatic Fever is an immunologic phenomenon caused by group A streptococcal (GAS) infection that affects various connective tissues in the body including the heart.

Table 5 Jones Criteria for rheumatic fever

Major manifestations	Minor manifestations
Carditis	Arthralgia
Polyarthritis	Fever
Chorea	Raised ESR rate or CRP
Erythema marginatum	Prolonged PR interval on EKG
Subcutaneous nodules	

Evidence of antecedent GAS infection
 1. Positive throat culture or rapid antigen test for GAS
 2. Other laboratory abnormalities (see Sect. 21.4)
Abbreviations: *CRP* c-reactive protein, *ESR* erythrocyte sedimentation rate, *GAS* group A streptococcus (Special Writing Group of the Committee on Rheumatic Fever *JAMA*. 1992)

21.1 General Considerations

Rheumatic fever (RF) is now relatively rare in the United States with treatment of Group A streptococcal (GAS) pharyngeal bacterial infections; however, a third of patients with RF do not recall symptoms of a previous throat infection. Multiple organ systems are affected by this immunogenic disorder such as the heart, joints, central nervous system, and dermis. Disorders of these four systems comprise the major criteria of the Jones system (see Table 5). The kidneys and lungs may also be affected. Cardiac symptoms are the most serious and specific manifestations of RF and can arise in 50–80% of patients. Joint pain is the most common symptom occurring in more than 80% of patients but is also the least specific. Arthritis is a major criteria and arthralgia is a minor criterion. The neurologic symptoms of Sydenham's chorea are a late manifestation, often 3 months after the pharyngitis and can be the initial manifestation. Chorea can occur in up to 30% of patients. The subcutaneous nodules and rash of erythema marginatum are relatively rare at 20% and 5%, respectively.

21.2 History

Usually about 3 weeks after the initial sore throat, multiple symptoms arise that often start with fevers. Chest pain indicative of pericarditis or pneumonitis may be present. Shortness of breath due to congestive heart failure (see above Sect. 4) is caused by valvular disease. Joint pain involves the large joints: shoulders, elbows, wrists, knees, and ankles. The joint pain is asymmetric, migratory, and transient. The constellation of neurologic symptoms called Sydenham's chorea is a complicated extrapyramidal disorder characterized by purposeless and involuntary movements and emotional lability. Difficulty writing, talking, and walking are initially reported which often causes the patient significant frustration. Epistaxis and abdominal pain resembling peritonitis is sometimes found.

21.3 Exam

Fever (a minor criteria) and tachycardia may be present. The holosystolic murmur of mitral regurgitation is the hallmark of the carditis of RF (a major criterion). The diastolic decrescendo murmur of aortic regurgitation may also be present. A friction rub of pericarditis may be present. Painless, firm, freely mobile subcutaneous nodules can be found in clusters on the extensor surfaces of knees, elbows and wrists. They can also be found over bony prominences, the dorsum of the foot, tendons, and the occipital area. The rash of erythema marginatum is macular irregular rashes with central clearing that spare the face.

21.4 Diagnostics

The EKG may show a variety of disturbances. The classic finding is the first-degree AV block (a minor criteria). QT prolongation may also be present. The urinalysis may show the pyuria and hematuria of glomerulonephritis, but this is not a defining criterion. Elevation of erythrocyte sedimentation rate (ESR) or C-reactive protein may be elevated (a minor criteria). A lab finding of GAS is necessary for diagnosis and can be historical (rapid strep or culture of GAS). Otherwise, subsequent testing for antigens and antibodies, such as ASO titers, streptococcal antigens and antibodies, and anti-DNAse B, is necessary.

Key Points
- Patients with rheumatic fever need to be hospitalized for monitoring and anti-inflammatory treatment.
- Rheumatic fever is defined by two major criteria and one minor or by one major and two minor criteria or four minor criteria (see Table 5).
- The murmur of mitral regurgitation is the most common cardiac manifestation which is a major criteria and joint pain is the most common symptom overall and is a minor criterion.
- Prolongation of the PR and fever are minor criteria.

Further Reading

Guidelines for the diagnosis of rheumatic fever. Jones Criteria, 1992 update. Special writing Group of the Committee on rheumatic fever, endocarditis and Kawasaki disease of the council on cardiovascular disease in the young. JAMA. 1992;268(15):20169–73.

Corrado D, Zorzi AC, M., et al. Relationship between arrhythmogenic right ventricular cardiomyopathy and Brugada syndrome: new insights from molecular biology and clinical implications. Circ Arrythm Electr. 2016;9:e003631.

Cydulka RK, Fitch MT, Joing SA, Wang VJ, Cline DM, Ma OJ, editors. Tintinalli's emergency medicine manual. 8th ed. New York: McGraw Hill; 2018.

Fauci AS, Braunwald E, Isselbacher KJ, Wilson JD, Martin JB, Kasper DL, Hauser SL, Longo DL. Harrison's principles of internal medicine. 14th ed. New York: McGraw Hill; 1998.

Friberg L, et al. Evaluation of risk stratification schemes for ischeamic stroke and bleeding in 182,678 patients with atrial fibrillation: the Swedish atrial fibrillation cohort study. Eur Heart J. 2012;10(33):1500–10.

Griffin BP, Topol EJ, editors. Manual of cardiovascular medicine. 2nd ed. Philadelphia, PA: Lippincott, Williams, and Wilkins; 2004.

Kline JA, Courtney DM, Kabrhel C, et al. Prospective multicenter evaluation of the pulmonary embolism rule-out criteria. J Thromb Haemost. 2008;6:772–80.

Lee Y, Habibzadeh MR, Movehed MR. Wellens syndrome or inverted U waves: a serious clinical condition needing immediate attention regardless of symptoms. Am J Med. 2021;134(11):1365–7.

Moumneh T, Sun B, et al. Identifying patients with low risk of acute coronary syndrome without troponin testing: validation of the hear score. Am J Med. 2021;134(4):499–506.

Prandoni P, Lensing AW, et al. Prevalence of pulmonary embolism among patients hospitalized for syncope. N Engl J Med. 2016;375:1524–31.

Six AJ, Backus BE, Kelder JC. Chest pain in the emergency room: value of the HEART score. Neth Heart J. 2008;16(6):191–6.

Surawicz B, Knilans TK. Chou's electrocardiography in clinical practice. London: W.B. Saunders; 2001.

Wells PS, Anderson DR, et al. Excluding pulmonary embolism at the bedside without diagnostic imaging: management of patients with suspected pulmonary embolism presenting to the emergency department by using a simple clinical model and d-dimer. Ann Inter Med. 2001;135(2):98–107.

Wells PS, Anderson DR, et al. Evaluation of D-dimer in the diagnosis of suspected deep-vein thrombosis. N Engl J Med. 2003;349(13):1227–35.

Infectious Disease

Taisiya Tumarinson and Cynthia Rivera

1 Introduction

Infections will be among the most common entities encountered in any clinical setting, and primary care is no exception. Virtually any infection can become severe and a monitored setting becomes advisable. Often, the need for emergency care is straightforward, but sometimes making that decision is elusive. This chapter will provide a review and some tips regarding how to navigate these clinical scenerios.

2 Sepsis and Toxic Shock

Severe sepsis and toxic shock are systemic syndromes characterized by hypotension and organ dysfunction usually due to a bacterial infection or bacterial toxin production, respectively.

T. Tumarinson (✉)
Miami Beach, FL, USA
e-mail: ttumarinson@gmail.com

C. Rivera
Department of Infectious Disease at FIU, Florida International University, Miami Beach, FL, USA
e-mail: cynrivera@yahoo.com

2.1 General Considerations

The incidence of sepsis originating in the community is hard to estimate, but the condition will be seen in an outpatient practice where same day acute visits are offered. Usually, gram negative or gram positive bacteria are the cause of sepsis; however, sepsis may be caused by any microorganism including viruses, fungi, or protozoa. The risk factors for sepsis are age > 65, obesity, immunosuppression due to organ transplantation and chemotherapy, and chronic conditions including diabetes. Cancer, malnutrition, and previous hospitalizations are other risk factors. Although the severe inflammatory response syndrome (SIRS) criteria (Table 1) are now less often used due to their non-specificity, they still provide a useful framework for evaluating patients who may need immediate care. The mortality of patients with the SIRS criteria, sepsis, and severe sepsis is 7%, 16%, and 20%, respectively. The management of potential sepsis in the office setting is based on prompt diagnosis and referral to the ED for the immediate initiation of IV fluids and IV antibiotics. Determining exact values for hypotension in the individual patient can be challenging, but the systemic inflammatory response (SIRS) criteria can be used as a guide. However, in chronically hypertensive patients, parameters for hypotension should be guided by the identification of blood pressures significantly lower than the patient's baseline. Toxic shock is a related syndrome caused by bacterial-derived toxins and can be caused by an infection of any source; however, it is often caused by skin infections from staphylococcus and streptococcus.

2.2 History

Altered mental status, fever, and/or chills may be reported. Shaking chills is an especially common symptom of bacteremia and should be noted. Sepsis, due to GU infections is the most common cause of sepsis. Urinary symptoms such as dysuria, urgency, and frequency often accompanied by systemic symptoms such as nausea or vomiting may be reported. Oliguria may be reported as renal perfusion decreases. Infections of the CNS, gastrointestinal infections, and pneumonia (see below) are other common causes of sepsis. Toxic shock syndromes have non-specific

Table 1 Systemic Inflammatory Response Syndrome (SIRS) (McClelland, H. and Moxon, A. *Nurs Times*. 2014)

Systemic Inflammatory Response Syndrome (SIRS)
Temperature > 38.3 °C, or <36 °C (>100.9 °F, or <96.8 °F)
Heart rate > 90 bpm
Respiratory rate > 20 breaths/min
White cell count <4 or >12 g/L
Blood glucose >140 mg/dL (in non-diabetic patients)
New altered mental state

Infectious Disease

symptoms such as malaise, arthralgias, cough, sore throat, rhinorrhea, and anorexia during early presentation. In staphylococcal toxic shock syndrome, a history of a bright red rash (erythroderma) described as a "painless sunburn" may be reported.

2.3 Exam

Hyperthermia or hypothermia may be present (Table 1). 90% of the time the heart rate is ≥90. Respiratory rate may be >20. The systolic blood pressure (SBP) is <90–100 mmHg or a 40 mmHg drop from the patient's baseline value. Orthostatic evaluation of blood pressure should be performed to assess for dehydration. Orthostasis is defined as a 20 mmHg drop in SBP or 10 mmHg drop in diastolic blood pressure (DBP) taken 30 s after going from a lying to a standing position. Assigning exact numbers to blood pressure is difficult to do in sepsis; and as in other shock states, the pulse pressure may be a useful indicator. The pulse pressure is the difference between the SBP and DBP. Pulse pressure often narrows prior to a frank decrease in the SBP. Other findings include crackles in the lungs (pneumonia or acute respiratory distress syndrome) and absent bowel sounds (ileus or abdominal infection). In toxic shock, the "painless sunburn" rash or desquamation may be seen. Vasculitic rashes (i.e., petechiae or purpura) can be seen with *N. meningitidis* and *S. pneumoniae*.

2.4 Diagnostics

There is no test for sepsis even in the inpatient setting. Hyperglycemia (glucose >140) in the absence of diabetes may be found on random measurement of glucose by glucometer. A urinalysis may show elevated specific gravity with a positive nitrites and leukocyte esterase. Microscopy will show bacteriuria with pyuria.

Key Points
- Hypotension or orthostasis and heart rate >90 combined with symptoms and/or signs of infection should be considered for referral to the ED.
- The primary care provider should be aware of SIRS criteria in ill-appearing patients; however, in suspected early sepsis, stringent compliance to these parameters is not necessary.
- Hypotension in hypertensive patients may be in the "normal" range.

3 Skin and Soft Tissue Infections

Soft tissue infections are common bacterial infections of the skin and underlying tissues.

3.1 General Considerations

Soft tissue infections are very common with 16 million ambulatory visits and 6 million ED visits annually for cellulitis which is the most common soft tissue infection. Most cases of cellulitis do not require hospitalization for IV antibiotics. Whether to refer patients with soft tissue infections to the ED depends not only on the severity of the infection but also on the patient's underlying comorbidities such as advancing age, peripheral vascular disease, and immunocompromised status including diabetes. Often, patients will need to be referred to the ED because they have failed outpatient therapy. Soft tissue infections requiring ED referral can be superficial (severe erysipelas), within the dermis (severe cellulitis) or in the subdermal tissues (necrotizing fasciitis). Erysipelas is a superficial cellulitis with associated lymphatic invasion caused by group A streptococcus (*S. pyogenes*) often associated with a port of entry. Necrotizing fasciitis may be mono-bacterial as in clostridial, staphylococcal, and streptococcal infections or may be polymicrobial, as often seen in diabetics. Clostridial infection (gas gangrene) is a true emergency requiring immediate surgery and IV antibiotics and carries a high mortality. Gas gangrene can be associated with trauma, recent surgery (especially hip surgery and surgery for fracture of long bones) and subcutaneous drug abuse (see Table 2). Gas gangrene can also be spontaneous, hematogenously spread from abdominal sources such as inflammatory bowel disease and colonic malignancies (including colonoscopic polypectomy). Cancers and chemotherapy especially with neutropenia is also associated with catastrophic clostridial infections. Necrotizing soft tissue infections are life-threatening but may appear at first to be deceptively benign. Thankfully, necrotizing soft tissue infections are rare with a global incidence of 10 cases per 100,000 persons but have a high mortality rate of 20–30%, especially if surgery is not performed within the first 24 h. In the USA, the most common risk factor for necrotizing skin infection is diabetes. Peripheral vascular disease, malnutrition, and alcoholism are also implicated. Soft tissue infections may be caused by skin flora and *Clostridium* spp., but also by gram

Table 2 Risk factors for necrotizing fasciitis and gas gangrene (*Clostridium perfringens*)

Risk Factors for Necrotizing Fasciitis	Risk Factors for Gas Gangrene
IVDA	Traumu
Diabetes	Orthopedic surgery (long bones)
Recent trauma	Subcutaneous drug use (a.k.a skin popping)
Recent surgery	Hematogenous (abdominal source, IBD, colon ca.)
PVD	Neutropenia/heme malignancy
Malnutrition	
Alcoholism	

Abbreviation: *IBD* inflammatory bowel disease

Infectious Disease

negative bacteria. One such bacteria, *Vibrio* spp. are associated with salt water and can cause severe explosive infections especially in those with liver disease and hemochromatosis.

3.2 History

A personal history of diabetes, peripheral vascular disease, IV drug abuse, and alcoholism is an important historical clue for risk of necrotizing fasciitis. A typical finding in necrotizing fasciitis is unexplained pain in a localized area of soft tissue with a fever. Necrotizing fasciitis is often associated with a port of entry and sometimes the trauma is minor. The presentation of necrotizing fasciitis is usually more abrupt than cellulitis. The typical history of necrotizing fasciitis is pain out of proportion to exam, especially described as deeper than the skin, whereas in cellulitis, the pain is more superficial. Numbness to light palpation of the skin due to damage of the subcutaneous nerves is reported however this is a late manifestation. Erysipelas has an associated burning sensation and the patient may report lymphadenopathy. Vibrio infections are associated with salt water exposure and often have intense pain around a fresh or old wound.

3.3 Exam

Fever may be present especially with erysipelas and *Vibrio* infections; however, the absence of a fever does not rule out a serious infection. Erysipelas is deep red, sharply demarcated and often associated with lymphangitis and lymphadenitis and often found on the unilateral lower extremity. In *Vibrio* infections, the infection often starts as erythematous patches and develops into ecchymosis, vesicles, and bullae. Hypotension may be found in necrotizing fasciitis, but is noted early in the disease process only 21% of the time. In necrotizing infections, the overlying skin is more of a brownish skin discoloration in contrast to the bright red of cellulitis, and bullae and serosanguinous discharge are often found. Tenderness to palpation can be quite severe unlike the mild to moderate pain associated with cellulitis. Crepitus, a crackling noise with palpation of the skin, is found in gas gangrene and is a late finding. Evidence of mild trauma can be found and sometimes hand trauma is found with infections of the shoulder or chest.

3.4 Diagnostics

Radiographs are of little value, being positive for gas in necrotizing fasciitis only 25% of the time.

Key Points
- Risk factors (especially diabetes) for severe cellulitis and necrotizing infection are similar and play a role in deciding patient disposition (see Table 2).
- Necrotizing skin infection may have fever, pain out of proportion to exam, bullae and purulent, serosanguinous discharge.
- If gas gangrene is suspected, EMS should be activated.

4 Septic Arthritis

Septic arthritis is a rare bacterial infection of the joint space that can affect nearly any joint.

4.1 General Considerations

The risk factors for septic arthritis are older age, diabetes, rheumatoid arthritis, and the history of a procedure such as joint surgery or intra-articular injection. Septic arthritis can be caused by hematogenous spread (often from IV drug use) or spread from a contiguous source such as cellulitis. The microorganisms are usually staphylococcus, streptococcus, or miscellaneous gram negative organisms. Disseminated gonorrheal infection (DGI) is often the cause in the younger population (age < 40). In the case of sickle cell disease, salmonella is common. Septic arthritis caused by hematogenous spread is oligo-articular 10–15% of the time and having more than one affected joint does not necessarily rule out the diagnosis. Oligo-articular septic arthritis may also be seen in rheumatoid arthritis and may resemble a typical disease flare. Nearly any joint can be affected, though large joints are most typically infected, especially the knee. The small joints are often infected by direct inoculation through a bite or trauma. In IV drug users, the appendicular skeleton is less frequently affected, and the spine, sternoclavicular joint, and sacroiliac joint are more commonly involved. In addition to antibiotics, drainage of the purulent material is also recommended. Arthroscopic drainage is associated with faster recovery.

4.2 History

A history of risk factors for gonorrheal infection should be sought in the younger population. Fevers and chills can be reported along with systemic symptoms such as malaise, but their absence does not rule out the diagnosis. In DGI, a preceding migratory tenosynovitis are a rash are common.

4.3 Exam

The hallmark examination finding of septic arthritis is pain with the passive movement of the joint of the severest nature. Restricted range of motion of the joint is common as is warmth and swelling of the joint. Near inability to move the joint due to pain is common. The rash of DGI is usually less than 25 lesions and starts as pinpoint red macules on the distal extremities, usually the extensor surfaces. Later, they may enlarge into vesicles and hemorrhagic bullae and evolve into necrotic centers (eschar) surrounded by an erythematous halo.

4.4 Diagnostics

The diagnosis is accomplished by a cell count with differential of synovial aspirate. Cultures of blood and synovial fluid performed in the hospital.

Key Points
- Septic arthritis is characterized by pain with passive movement of the severest nature, often resulting in near immobility of the joint. These patients require joint aspiration and IV antibiotics.
- If findings of a possible disseminated gonorrheal infection are found, the patient requires IV antibiotics.

5 Osteomyelitis

Osteomyelitis is a bacterial infection in the bones either resulting from infections in the surrounding tissues or hematogenous spread. Osteomyelitis can be classified as acute or chronic, and in either case, long-term antibiotics are required.

6 Contiguous Osteomyelitis

6.1 General Considerations

Approximately several hundred thousand cases of osteomyelitis occur in the U.S. annually. Contiguous osteomyelitis occurs in patients with skin ulceration or breakdown from various etiologies. The most common type of contiguous osteomyelitis is seen in diabetic patients with open foot wounds (i.e., the diabetic foot ulcer). Peripheral vascular disease (PVD) and extremes of age also contribute to the risk of diabetic foot ulcers. Other common causes of contiguous osteomyelitis are sacral decubitus ulcers. The infection in these two types of ulcers is usually polymicrobial and difficult to treat, typically requiring long-term antibiotics and intensive wound care. In addition to these common causes, essentially any bone can become infected from surrounding tissues. The temporal bones can develop contiguous osteomyelitis resulting in a life-threatening condition called malignant otitis externa. Any bone of the peripheral skeleton is also susceptible, especially in patients with joint replacements. The microorganisms involved in prosthetic joint infections are most commonly staphylococcal species.

6.2 History

The history of the diabetic foot with osteomyelitis is non-specific and is often complicated by concomitant neuropathy. The symptoms of cellulitis are sometimes present. Systemic symptoms of fever, chills, and malaise may be present in any form of contiguous osteomyelitis and aid in diagnosis.

6.3 Exam

Foot ulcers due to diabetes and sometimes PVD will have a chronic wound which may be tender and have purulent drainage. Visible bone may be present in the wound bed. Probing the wound or sinus tract with a sterile instrument and reaching bone (positive probe to bone test) has a high likelihood of being osteomyelitis. Any foot wound >2 cm is at high risk of being osteomyelitis.

6.4 Diagnostics

X-rays are cost effective but have lower sensitivity and specificity at around 50% and 70%, respectively, in the case of diabetic ulcer. MRI is the test of choice with sensitivity and specificity around 80–90% as early as 3–5 days after onset of osteomyelitis. Elevated inflammatory markers have excellent sensitivity for prosthetic joint infections (>90%) but have somewhat less specificity (70–80%).

Key Points
- Diabetic foot ulcers 2 cm or larger are at risk for osteomyelitis.
- Patients with a positive probe to bone test are likely to have osteomyelitis.
- Patients with non-healing foot ulcers should be co-managed with a podiatrist who can proceed with bone biopsy, debridement, or amputation if necessary.

7 Vertebral Osteomyelitis

Vertebral osteomyelitis is a rare bone infection of the vertebral column.

7.1 General Considerations

About 17,000 cases of vertebral osteomyelitis occur annually. Risk factors are age >65, diabetes, immunocompromised state including chronic steroid use and chronic kidney disease. Lumbar spine osteomyelitis is the most common location and can originate from a urinary tract infection and IV drug use. Endocarditis is also often associated with vertebral osteomyelitis. In those patients from endemic areas, tuberculosis (TB) can infect the spine, a condition known as Pott's disease. Direct inoculation can also occur postoperatively and from epidural injections. Vertebral osteomyelitis can also occur hematogenously or contiguously from infections in contiguous locations. Retropharyngeal abscess, empyema, psoas muscle abscess, and decubitus ulcers are reported to infect the vertebral bones. Paraspinal abscesses and spinal epidural abscess can occur (see chapter "Neurology"). The most common site of vertebral osteomyelitis is the lumbar spine (58%) followed by thoracic (30%) and cervical (12%).

7.2 History

Fevers are reported 35–60% of the time. 90% of the time there is back or neck pain reported, often worse at night and unrelieved by position or medications. Neurologic symptoms may be reported (25%), usually in association with epidural abscess (see chapter "Neurology").

7.3 Exam

Fever may be present. Tenderness directly over the affected vertebra is often present.

7.4 Diagnostics

Leukocytosis is an unreliable finding; however, the inflammatory markers, ESR and CRP, have a very good sensitivity for this disorder (99%), less so when indolent pathogens are causative agents of disease. Note that inflammatory markers also have a very high sensitivity for epidural abscess.

Key Points
- Fevers and point tenderness over an affected vertebra are concerning for osteomyelitis especially in a patient with risk factors.
- Inflammatory markers are useful in unclear cases, particularly for trending efficacy of therapeutics.

8 Pyelonephritis

Pyelonephritis is a kidney infection, the upper most part of the urinary tract.

8.1 General Considerations

Pyelonephritis is common with more than 500,000 cases occurring annually. This infection generally requires initial treatment with intravenous antibiotics followed by a transition to oral agents. Pregnant women, men with prostatic hypertrophy, the elderly, and those with pre-existing comorbidities such as diabetes and immunosuppression are most susceptible to pyelonephritis. Pyelonephritis usually occurs as an ascending infection, starting out as a UTI. The most common pathogen is *E. coli* (80%) with other pathogens *Proteus*, *Pseudomonas*, *Klebsiella*, and *S. saprophyticus* comprising the remainder. A history of urologic procedures, stones, anatomic abnormalities of the urinary tract, and immunocompromised states, including diabetes, place the patient at risk for an abscess. Patients who do not respond after 72 h of therapy need an evaluation for an underlying obstruction or abscess.

8.2 History

Up to 20% of patients with pyelonephritis do not have urinary symptoms, elderly patients in particular. In the elderly with pyelonephritis, other symptoms such as abdominal pain, weakness, and altered mental status are often seen. The clinical distinction between upper and lower urinary tract infection is generally straightforward with flank pain, fever, chills, nausea with or without vomiting being the hallmarks of pyelonephritis.

8.3 Exam

Fever is often present along with nausea and vomiting. Hypotension and tachycardia are common and a cause for concern. Unilateral costovertebral tenderness is often found with pyelonephritis.

8.4 Diagnostics

Urinalysis should be abnormal with the presence of leukocytes with or without nitrites and erythrocytes. Microscopy reveals pyuria. The urinalysis is of less utility when there is glucose or increased levels of protein in the urine. A culture with susceptibility needs to be obtained when dealing with suspected pyelonephritis. If a patient fails to improve, an abdominal ultrasound or radiograph should be obtained to evaluate for the presence of an abscess or free air. Emphysematous pyelonephritis is a lethal condition that can occur in diabetics or the immunocompromised.

Key Points
- The presence of intractable vomiting and/or hemodynamic instability require inpatient admission.
- Care should be taken with pregnant women as they become septic 20% of the time.
- Emphysematous pyelonephritis, defined by free air in the perinephric space, or an abscess is an emergency requiring ED referral, often found in immunocompromised patients including diabetes, patients with nephrolithiasis, and patients with unresolving pyelonephritis.

9 Infective Endocarditis

Infective endocarditis (IE) is an infection of the lining of the heart that is usually on the valves and is caused by a variety of organisms.

9.1 General Considerations

Approximately 17,000 cases of endocarditis (IE) occur each year. Three strong risk factors associated with IE are prosthetic heart valves, hemodialysis, and previous IE. Structural heart disease is present in approximately 75% of patients with IE. Structural lesions of the valves can be acquired (i.e., rheumatic heart disease, Aortic sclerosis) or congenital (hypertrophic cardiomyopathy, bicuspid aortic valve, etc.). Mitral valve prolapse has a strong association but only when accompanied by regurgitation of the valve. Other risk factors for endocarditis are age >60 years, male sex, injection drug use, poor dentition or current dental infection, and immunosuppression. *S. aureus* (especially seen in acute IE in IV drug users and in patients with prosthetic valves) is the leading cause of IE in the industrialized world. Viridans group streptococci, and enterococci are also common. *Streptococcus gallolyticus* (formerly *Streptococcus bovis*) endocarditis is rare and is associated with abnormalities of the colonic mucosa, usually seen with colon cancer or inflammatory bowel disease. Criteria have been devised to define patients with a definitive, possible, or rejected diagnosis of IE (see Table 3).

Table 3 Duke's Criteria for Infective endocarditis (Li, J.S., Sexton, D.J. et al. *Clin infect Dis.* 2000)

Major Criteria
Positive blood culture
• Typical organism from two cultures
• Persistent positive blood cultures taken >12 h apart
• Three or more positive cultures taken over >1 h
Endocardial involvement
• Positive echocardiographic findings of vegetations
• New valvular regurgitation
Minor Criteria
Predisposing valvular or cardiac abnormality
Intravenous drug use
Fever ≥38 °C (100.4 °F)
Embolic phenomenon
Vasculitic phenomenon
Blood cultures suggestive-organism grown but not achieving major criteria
Suggestive echocardiographic findings
Definite endocarditis: two major, or one major and three minor, or five minor
Possible endocarditis: one major and one minor, or three minor

9.2 History

Onset can be abrupt and severe or it can be insidious with a subacute presentation. Fever is present in 80–90% of patients. Non-specific symptoms such as headache, myalgias, arthralgias, abdominal pain, dyspnea, malaise, and night sweats may be present. Various symptoms associated with complications can be found. Examples include vertebral osteomyelitis and septic emboli to various organs including the brain and lungs with an associated disruption of their function.

9.3 Exam

A cardiac murmur, either pre-existing or new, is present 85% of the time. Petechiae are present 20–40% of the time in subacute IE, usually found on the extremities, palate, or conjunctivae. Another finding that is rare but specific for subacute IE is Osler nodes, tender subcutaneous violaceous nodules on the pads of fingers and toes. In acute IE, Janeway lesions, nontender, red macules on the palms and soles can be found.

9.4 Diagnostics

The urinalysis may show leukocytes and erythrocytes found in glomerulonephritis. The EKG may show various blocks including first degree AV block indicating extension of the vegetation into the conduction system. Blood cultures should be positive, even in an afebrile patient, but can be negative 5–15% of the time in subacute endocarditis with fastidious organisms. Normocytic anemia may be present; CRP and ESR are usually elevated. CRP is elevated more than 90% of the time. A rheumatoid factor or RPR may be positive.

Key Points
- Endocarditis is a diagnosis that cannot be missed in a patient with a fever and cardiac murmur, especially if the murmur is new.
- Risk factors for endocarditis include IV drug use and those with prosthetic valves.
- A CRP is elevated more than 90% of the time.
- The Dukes criteria have been developed which outline possible and definite endocarditis (see Table 3).

10 Pneumonia

Pneumonia is a common infection of the lung parenchyma often resulting in hypoxia and hypotension with ensuing morbidity and mortality.

10.1 General Considerations

Pneumonia is a common complication of respiratory infection resulting in millions of visits each year to healthcare settings. The risk factors for developing severe community acquired pneumonia (CAP) are chronic obstructive pulmonary disease, diabetes mellitus, renal disease, congestive heart failure, stroke, and coronary heart disease (Table 4).

Pneumonia is divided into typical and atypical causes. Typical pneumonia most often causes lobar (unilateral) lung infection, classically caused by *Pneumococcus* spp. Atypical pneumonias are caused by a variety of organisms, both bacterial and

Table 4 Risk factors for severe pneumonia

Risk factors for severe pneumonia
COPD
Diabetes
Renal disease
Cancer
Coronary artery disease
Congestive heart failure
Stroke
Male sex

Abbreviation: *COPD* chronic obstructive pulmonary disease

viral, and commonly cause bilateral lung infections. Atypical bacterial causes are *Mycoplasma, Legionella, H. influenza, C. pneumoniae,* and *M. catarrhalis*. The decision to refer the patient to the ED depends on comorbidities, age, and vital signs. Several decision rules have been developed for evaluation in the ED such as the CURB-65 and the pneumonia severity index (PSI). The CURB-65 rule is simple and identifies confusion, uremia, elevated respiratory rate, hypotension, and age >65 as high risk for mortality and indication for admission. The PSI is much more detailed and cumbersome; however, additional risk factors for poor outcome include male sex, cancer, congestive heart failure, stroke, renal and liver disease and are noted to be part of the calculus in this decision tool. The CRB-65 rule has been adapted from the CURB-65 to guide clinicians in the outpatient setting (see Table 5), and patients without these factors are considered lower risk. The CRB-65 rule and PSI are meant to inform the clinician but do not replace clinical judgment. The presence of COPD and low oxygen saturation (<92% as a general guideline in non-COPD patients) are other risk factors for decompensation that should be considered. It should be noted that cases of pneumonia are often complicated with accompanying cardiac issues such as myocardial infarction, congestive heart failure, and arrhythmias.

10.2 History

Fever, cough, fatigue, and shortness of breath are typically reported. Often, the cough is productive of sputum which is sometimes purulent. Diarrhea can be reported with legionella. Up to 20% of patients have other gastrointestinal symptoms such as nausea and vomiting. Other non-specific symptoms such as headache, myalgias, and arthralgias may be reported.

10.3 Exam

Adventitious lung sounds such as crackles, rhonchi, and wheezing may be present, unilaterally (lobar pneumonia) or bilaterally. A bulging tympanic membrane (bullous myringitis) can be seen with mycoplasma pneumonia.

Table 5 The CRB-65 score for evaluating severe pneumonia (Ebell, M. and Walsh, M. *J Gen Intern Med.* 2019)

CRB-65	Score	Mortality	Recommendation
Each risk factor scores one point with a maximum score of 4 Confusion of new onset Respiratory rate > 30/min or greater Blood pressure < 90 mmHg systolic or <65 mmHg diastolic Age > 65 years	0	0.5%	Low risk
	1–2	5.1%	Moderate risk
	3–4	18.9%	High risk

10.4 Diagnostics

A chest radiograph is recommended, but it is limited by relatively low sensitivity. If the radiograph is abnormal, multilobar infiltrates are a risk factor for deterioration.

Key Points
- The CRB-65 details some notable causes for ED referral (see Table 5).
- A low oxygen saturation (<92%) and risk factors as detailed above are also part of the calculus.
- The patient's social status should also be assessed as borderline patients treated in the community will need support for monitoring in the home.

11 Tuberculosis

Tuberculosis (TB) is an infection of tissues (usually the lungs) with *Mycobacterium tuberculosis* that requires isolation during the infective stage.

11.1 General Considerations

TB is the second leading cause of infectious disease death worldwide and is still a cause of significant morbidity and mortality in the U.S. with about 10,000 cases reported to the CDC in 2015. The main reason for the maintenance of these levels of TB in the U.S. is due to the rise of HIV and immigration. TB may also be contracted by travelers to endemic countries (see Sect. 14). Other risk factors for TB are living or working in prisons, shelters, or long-term care facilities, and abuse of drugs or alcohol. Transmission occurs through airborne and droplet spread from a patient who is afflicted with pulmonary tuberculosis. A person with exposure to *M. tuberculosis* but without symptoms and with a clear chest X-ray is considered to have latent tuberculosis infection (LTBI) if they have a positive tuberculin skin test (TST) or interferon-gamma release assay (IGRA). Reactivation occurs in approximately 10% of patients with LTBI and is more likely to occur during periods of immunosuppression or waning immunity (i.e., aging). Therefore, patients with latent TB are treated according to current guidelines. When there is a high suspicion of TB, the patient should be masked immediately and sent to the hospital for further testing and isolation. Despite being primarily a respiratory illness, extrapulmonary manifestations are common (30% of the time) and can affect almost any organ system. Painless lymphadenitis (i.e., scrofula in the cervical lymph nodes) is an example. Extrapulmonary TB is even more common in HIV patients (60–70%). A clinical pearl regarding when to include TB in your working diagnosis is when a patient is not improving after treatment for community acquired pneumonia (CAP).

11.2 History

Fever, cough, pleuritic chest pain, and shortness of breath represent active pulmonary infection usually seen in children. Reactivation (from latent TB) often presents subacutely with malaise, cough, hemoptysis, low grade fevers, and night sweats with weight loss. Reactivation occurs in approximately 10% of patients with latent TB and is more likely to occur as immunity wanes (i.e. during aging).

11.3 Exam

Fever may be present with active infection. Low grade fever is often seen with reactivation. The pulmonary exam may reveal adventitious sounds such as crackles, wheezing and rhonchi; however, the pulmonary exam is often normal.

11.4 Diagnostics

Active TB can cause infiltrates, mediastinal lymphadenopathy, and effusions in isolation or in combination on chest radiography. Reactivation classically presents with lesions in the upper lobes or superior segments of lower lobes. Cavitation, calcification, scarring, and atelectasis are also found in reactivation. Both normal and immunosuppressed patients (i.e., HIV) can have normal or atypical chest radiographs. Asymptomatic patients, incidentally, found to have latent TB, may have scarring, volume loss, and calcification which does not imply infectivity.

Key Points
- Patients with risk factors for TB and typical symptoms should be masked and referred to the ED to rule out TB.
- TB should be considered in patients clinically diagnosed with community acquired pneumonia but not improving on antibiotics.
- In lower risk cases, patients can be referred for a chest radiograph to look for typical findings associated with TB.
- A normal radiograph does not rule out TB.

12 Cases of Immunosuppression

12.1 Human Immunodeficiency Virus (HIV)

HIV infection may lead to immunosuppression by disabling the cellular immunity of the patent.

12.1.1 General Considerations

Approximately 1.2 million individuals live with HIV in the US, categorizing the US as a low prevalence setting. Risk factors in the U.S. include IV drug use, men who have sex with men (MSM), sex workers, transgendered individuals, and prisoners. HIV targets and destroys T-helper (CD4+) cells causing profound immunosuppression. Great strides have been made in HIV research and treatment. For patients taking antiretroviral therapy (ART), HIV has become a chronic manageable disease with near normal life expectancy, particularly when treatment is initiated within 6 months of seroconversion. Current recommendations are to start ART as soon as possible following diagnosis. If untreated, HIV causes acquired immunodeficiency syndrome (AIDS). AIDS is diagnosed by the presence of an opportunistic infection (OI) or a CD4+ count below 200 cells/µL. Today, OIs due to AIDS are less common due to ART; however, in some settings, OIs with mycobacterial, fungal, protozoan, and viral organisms are still encountered (Table 6). On occasion, OIs can present as the initial presentation of HIV. Testing includes CD4+ counts, HIV RNA PCR, and genotypic/phenotypic assays. Suppression of viral load is the cornerstone of HIV management with the goal of patients achieving undetectable viral loads. As long as viral load remains <200 copies/mL, the risk of sexually transmitting HIV is negligible. CD4+ counts can vary depending on recent illnesses or inflammatory processes which can cause consumption. Latent infections and malignancies can be reactivated upon the initiation of ART. This is more common in patients started on therapy with a lower CD4 count. Patients started on ART whose health deteriorates should be referred for admission due to suspicion for Immune Reconstitution Inflammatory Syndrome (IRIS). Symptoms are typically non-specific and include fever, lymphadenopathy, or symptoms specific to the primary infection that is reactivated. A closely monitored setting is advisable for rapid initiation of necessary treatment, supportive care and observation. Usually most acute medical conditions in patients living with HIV are managed in close coordination with an infectious disease specialist, especially in patients whose disease is not controlled and for whom resistance is suspected.

12.1.2 History

Fever, dry cough, and shortness of breath can be associated with *Pneumocystis jiroveci* pneumonia (PJP) and tuberculosis (TB) (see Table 6). Fever and headache and other neurologic symptoms can present subacutely in Toxoplasma encephalitis and Cryptococcal meningitis (see Table 6). Subacute watery diarrhea and abdominal cramping are associated with cryptosporidiosis (see Table 6). Lactic acidosis in the HIV patient can present with vague complaints initially. Examples include fatigue, malaise, nausea with or without vomiting, abdominal pain, and shortness of breath (see Table 7). Eye symptoms are associated with CMV retinitis, zoster keratitis and retinitis, and herpes simplex keratitis.

Table 6 Opportunistic infections in human immunodeficiency virus (HIV)

	Opportunistic infection	Cause	CD4 cells/mm³	Symptoms	Diagnosis	Special considerations
Lung	Pneumocystis pneumonia (PJP)	*Pneumocystis jiroveci* (fungus)	<200	*Cough, fever*, dyspnea, tachypnea	Hypoxemia, chest radiograph: diffuse bilateral interstitial infiltrates (may appear normal in early disease)	Normal CT has high negative predictive value
	Tuberculosis (TB)	*Mycobacterium tuberculosis*	<200	*Cough, Fever*, night sweats, weight loss, lymphadenitis, osteomyelitis	Chest radiograph may appear normal or atypical (with low CD 4 count no predilection for upper lobes), anemia	Extrapulmonary presentations increase with degree of immunodeficiency
Brain	Toxoplasma encephalitis	*Toxoplasma gondii* (protozoan)	<50	*Headache, Fever*, confusion, focal deficits	CT of brain plus contrast	Sources: cat feces, undercooked meat, raw shellfish.
	Cryptococcal meningitis	*Cryptococcus neoformans* (encapsulated yeast)	<100	*Headache, Fever*, subacute meningitis	Lumbar puncture with high opening pressure. CSF analysis for antigen	Meningeal symptoms, photophobia, occur in only 25% of patients
Abdomen	Cryptosporidiosis	*Cryptosporidium* (protozoan)	<100	*Abdominal pain*, subacute watery diarrhea	Stool oocyst evaluation	Severity can range from asymptomatic to cholera-like
	MAC disease	*Mycobacterium avium intracellulare*	<50	*Abdominal pain, Fever*, night sweats, weight loss, diarrhea	Anemia, elevated alk phos, lymphadenopathy and enlarged liver and spleen on CT of chest and abdomen	ART will lead to IRIS, which is clinically indistinguishable from active MAC infection

Abbreviations: *Alk. phos.* alkaline phosphatase, *ART* active retroviral therapy, *CT* computed tomography, *IRIS* immune reconstitution inflammatory syndrome, *PJP* Pneumocystis jiroveci pneumonia

12.1.3 Exam

Typical findings associated with an abnormal pulmonary exam can be seen with PJP and TB. Altered mental status and focal neurologic deficits are seen in encephalitis and meningitis (see Table 6).

Key Points
- Acutely symptomatic patients with known HIV are usually managed in close coordination with an ID specialist.
- Opportunistic infections occur (see Table 6) and can be the initial presentation.
- The febrile, non-specific condition of Immune Reconstitution Syndrome (IRIS) can occur after initiation of ART and requires hospitalization.
- Lactic acidosis can present with subtle symptoms in patients taking (nucleoside reverse transcriptase inhibitors (NRTI) therapy (see Table 7).
- Hepatitis can occur with all ART (see Table 7).
- Pancreatitis and hyperglycemia can be caused by protease inhibitors (see Table 7).

12.2 Transplant Patients

Transplant patients are on immunosuppressive medications and have a decreased ability to fight infections. Immunosuppressive agents also mask the usual signs and symptoms of infections. They are susceptible to opportunistic infections in addition to common pathogens.

Table 7 Side effects of active retroviral therapy (ART)

Symptoms	Medicine	Condition	Location of Pain	Other findings	Laboratories
Abdominal pain, nausea and vomiting	NRTI	Lactic acidosis	Generalized	*Mild*: fatigue, edema/ascites, dyspnea *Severe*: multi-organ failure, pancreatitis, pancytopenia	CBC, CMP (bicarb), lipase 2–3× > normal range
	All classes	Hepatitis	Right upper quadrant	Fatigue, pruritus, jaundice	AST, or ALT 3–5× > normal range
	PI	Diabetes, hyperglycemia, DKA	Generalized	Polydipsia, polyuria, polyphagia, weight loss	Bicarb, anion gap
		Pancreatitis	Upper abdomen	Fever	Lipase 2–3× > normal range

Abbreviations: *DKA* diabetic ketoacidosis, *NRTI* nucleoside reverse transcriptase inhibitors, *PI* protease inhibitors

12.2.1 General Considerations

Approximately 35,000 solid organ transplants occur annually with renal transplant being most common. Hematopoietic cell transplants are slightly less common with around 20,000 performed every year. Emergency room visits are common in this population, with approximately 40% of transplant recipients needing an ED visit within the first year. Iatrogenic immunosuppression is required to prevent rejection of the transplanted tissue which makes transplant patients particularly vulnerable to infections. Infections are bacterial, fungal and viral. Unusual organisms that are not commonly seen in immunocompetent patients are referred to as opportunistic infections (OI). Transplant patients receive prophylaxis against *Pneumocystis jiroveci* pneumonia (PJP), cytomegalovirus, and various fungi. Some also receive prophylaxis for *Mycobacterium Avium Intracellulare* (MAI). Along with the risk of infection, patients are also at risk for death due to cardiovascular disease and renal failure (even in non-kidney solid organ transplants). Therefore, complaints of chest pain or dyspnea should prompt referral to the ED to evaluate for ACS. Serial monitoring of renal function is also recommended.

12.2.2 History

Infections can present in a more subtle manner than in immunocompetent patients. Fever may be less prominent or absent. Lymphadenopathy may be present due to various infections such as toxoplasmosis or Epstein–Barr virus. Ophthalmic symptoms may represent cytomegalovirus (CMV) or toxoplasmosis, and these patients should see an ophthalmologist on the same day. Sinusitis symptoms and headache may represent mucormycosis. A mild cough or scant diarrhea can mask a serious infection from a variety of organisms. CMV pneumonia is a common and serious illness. Right upper quadrant pain representing bile leaks is common in liver transplant patients. Diarrhea is often caused by *C. difficile*.

12.2.3 Exam

Fever may be absent. Altered mental status, sometimes subtle, can arise from a number of infectious sources. The nares should be closely inspected to investigate for mucormycosis, a potentially devastating infection. Strongyloidiasis and Chagas disease (transmitted through infected organs or via reactivation due to immunosuppression) may present with cutaneous manifestations.

12.2.4 Diagnostics

Pyuria may be absent on urine studies despite a urinary tract infection. Chest imaging may be falsely negative in the setting of pneumonia.

Key Points
- Transplant recipients are vulnerable to a variety of opportunistic infections and their care should be in close coordination with their transplant team.
- The presentation of serious infections in these patients is often less pronounced in immunocompetent patients.

13 Neutropenic Fever

Neutropenic fever is defined as a single measurement of 38.5 °C (101.3 °F) or a continuous measurement above 38 °C (100.4 °F) for 1 h in the presence of an absolute neutrophil count of 500–1000 cells/µL. It occurs in the presence of low neutrophils associated with chemotherapy, hematopoietic cell transplants, and some hematologic malignancies.

13.1 General Considerations

Neutropenic fever is a common oncologic emergency with a mortality of 5–20% depending on age and comorbidities. Mortality can reach 50% if the patient presents in shock, so early recognition and treatment of neutropenic fever is paramount. Broad spectrum IV antibiotics should be started within the hour for neutrophil counts <500 and the presence of fever. Neutrophil counts typically reach a nadir 10–15 days after the last dose of chemotherapy. Most patients have been instructed by their oncologist to report to the ED in the presence of a fever for blood work during this critical period for evidence of infection. Neutropenic patients are susceptible to typical infections seen in the community as well as infections caused by unusual pathogens due to their decreased immunity.

13.2 History

Fever is usually the presenting complaint. On the rare occasion that an infection is readily identifiable, patients can complain of dysuria, diarrhea, cough, or a rash.

13.3 Exam

The exam as well as the history may be less convincing than in the immunocompetent patient. Patients should be given early empiric broad spectrum antibiotics and antifungals, at least for a short duration based only on a presumptive diagnosis.

Key Point
- Patients with a single measurement of 38.5 °C (101.3 °F) or a measured fever of 38 °C (100.4 °F) continuously for an hour are at risk for neutropenia and should be referred to the ED.

14 The Febrile Traveler

Febrile Travelers are patients returning from trips that may have developed infections endemic to their travel locales. Occasionally, these infections are potentially life-threatening and require hospitalization.

14.1 General Considerations

Many of the infections discussed here have variable virulence, often causing minor infections and do not necessarily cause serious disease or even come to medical attention. Diagnosing a patient who has become ill after recent travel can be very challenging. Infections can be contracted upon return in the patient's native environment or be endemic to their travel destinations. As a general rule, most infections attributable to travel occur within 1 month of leaving the destination. A sexual history from all travelers is appropriate to assess for acute HIV for which many rapid tests are insensitive. Travelers returning from tropical locations are vulnerable to arthropod-borne virus (arboviruses); typically, the vector is the mosquito. Malaria is the infection that causes the most morbidity and mortality and is the number one concern, especially in travelers returning from West Africa. Malaria is a protozoan infection from *Plasmodium* spp. spread from the *Anopheles* mosquito. Four other infections discussed here are also arboviruses from mosquitos. Yellow fever, Dengue, and Zika are RNA flaviviruses spread mainly by the *Aedes aegypti* mosquito while chikungunya is a RNA togavirus, also spread by *Aedes aegypti*.

After malaria, enteric fever, commonly contracted in Asia, is the most common cause of mortality. Rickettsial diseases can be found in international travelers, including scrub typhus (Asia) and Rocky Mountain spotted fever (Mexico and South America). However, Rocky Mountain spotted fever is generally found in the U.S. and has been reported in every state. Leptospirosis is commonly a traveler's disease in those who have had freshwater or animal exposure.

In addition to the clinical variables of the patient's presentation, the patient's entire itinerary must also be considered, and the geographic range of the specific organism will be briefly discussed. A traveler's fever can have numerous etiologies, and this chapter is not an exhaustive list. In this regard, the complexity of cases of febrile travelers are such that online support is available to clinicians as decision tools (www.fevertravel.ch). The Centers for Disease Control (CDC) also has support available to clinicians for diagnosis and treatment such as the CDC malaria hotline.

The most deadly traveler's tropical diseases are falciparum malaria (77%) and enteric fever (18%), but rare fatalities have also been reported with rickettsial diseases (Mediterranean spotted fever, murine typhus, and scrub typhus) and melioidosis. Increased age is associated with risk of morbidity and mortality due to infections, and diseases of travel are no exception. The following infections may be distinguished by the presence or absence of a rash as a useful clinical distinction. However, not all patients with those infections having a characteristic rash will present with that rash.

15 Fever Without a Rash

15.1 *Malaria*

Malaria is an infection by the protozoan spp. *Plasmodium* spread by the *Anopheles* mosquito.

15.1.1 General Considerations

Malaria should ALWAYS be on the differential diagnosis in a patient with fever and recent travel to an endemic area. Approximately 2000 cases of malaria are diagnosed in the US annually. The overwhelming number of these cases are represented by returning travelers. On rare occasions, malaria can also be transmitted from blood transfusions, vertical transmission, and local mosquito-borne transmission.

Malaria is widespread among 80 countries and is the most common infection endemic to many areas of the world including sub-Saharan Africa, Central and South America, Indian subcontinent, Southeast Asia, the middle east, and Oceania. Travelers to sub-Saharan Africa have the greatest risk of getting malaria and dying from it. More than 50% of cases in the U.S. arise from travel to Africa, and 22% of malaria cases in the U.S. are reported as severe. *Plasmodium falciparum* is the most common species found in U.S. patients and is the most virulent species of the *Plasmodium* genus. *Plasmodium Falciparum* is the sole species that causes the syndrome of Blackwater Fever, characterized by massive hemolysis, jaundice, and renal failure. In its life cycle, malaria infects hepatocytes which rupture and release merozoites. These merozoites from the ruptured hepatocytes in turn infect erythrocytes which then also rupture resulting in jaundice and hemolytic anemia respectively. The typical incubation period of malaria is 1–4 weeks. In cases of *P. ovale* and *P. vivax*, the infection can remain dormant in the liver from 3 weeks to a year or longer. This can cause relapsing infections when the patient is infected with these two species.

15.1.2 History

Fevers may be reported, often in regular cycles, reflecting intermittent infection and rupture of red blood cells. However, this pattern is absent particularly early in the infection with *P. falciparum*. Classically, the cycles of fever are followed by profuse diaphoresis and exhaustion. Other features of malaria are non-specific and include headache, abdominal pain, nausea, vomiting, shortness of breath, arthralgias, and myalgias. Severe malaria symptoms include neurologic symptoms, seizures, confusion, and shortness of breath.

15.1.3 Exam

Fever may be present. Pallor may indicate severe anemia. Scleral icterus and hepatosplenomegaly may be present with significant hemolysis. In severe malaria, crackles may be indicative of pulmonary edema.

15.1.4 Diagnostics

Patients with a high risk of malaria should be referred to the ED for diagnostic workup. Thin and thick smears from the peripheral blood should be prepared. Once the presence of the parasite is confirmed, the species can also be identified and parasite density calculated. Non-specific laboratory findings include normocytic anemia, low platelet counts, as well as elevated ESR and CRP. Unconjugated bilirubin is elevated in jaundiced patients indicating hemolysis.

Key Points
- An unexplained febrile illness in a patient returning from an endemic region should raise concern for malaria.
- Patients should be referred to the ED for laboratory testing.
- Most patients with *P. falciparum* and *P. knowlesi* need to be admitted and observed for disease progression.
- The CDC's malaria hotline is available for consultations (1-800-232-4636).

15.2 Yellow Fever

Yellow fever is an arthropod-borne RNA flavivirus which causes jaundice giving the syndrome its name.

15.2.1 General Considerations

The infection is endemic to Africa and Central and South American countries where it is relatively common. The World Health Organization estimates that there are 200,000 cases of clinical disease and 30,000 deaths from yellow fever annually.

Approximately 15% of patients get moderate to severe disease. The incubation period is approximately 3–6 days.

15.2.2 History

Sudden onset of high fever is reported along with headache, vertigo, and nausea with or without vomiting. Pain is described in the neck, back, and legs. A bleeding diathesis with epistaxis and gingival bleeding may be present. In the beginning, the presentation can be confused with malaria, dengue, and leptospirosis infection. A brief period where the fever abates for approximately 2 days is followed by progression of the illness. Later neurologic symptoms such as delirium and agitation can ensue along with progression of bleeding to melena and hematemesis. Yellow fever is clinically indistinguishable from malaria and referral to the ED is indicated for diagnostic testing and observation.

15.2.3 Exam

Fever is present and may be quite high. A paradoxical bradycardia with the fever known as Faget's sign is often present. Conjunctival injection is often seen. Jaundice is characteristic.

15.2.4 Diagnostics

Virus specific immunoglobulin IgM and IgG are available on serologic testing. Vaccination history is important as IgM can persist for years following vaccination. PCR testing is also available. However, by the time symptoms are recognized, the viral DNA is undetectable. The CDC has a hotline for assistance in diagnosing yellow fever.

Key Point
- Yellow fever has the characteristics of conjunctival injection, jaundice, and a bleeding diathesis which often heralds severe infection. The diagnosis is clinical and treatment is only supportive even in severe cases.

15.3 *Leptospirosis*

Leptospirosis is a zoonotic infection caused by various members of the Leptospira species (spirochetes). It has clinical features similar to yellow fever except it can develop rashes that generally last <24 h.

15.3.1 General Considerations

The true incidence of leptospirosis is unknown, but it is thought that perhaps one million moderate to severe cases occur world-wide with a 10% mortality rate. Most leptospirosis infections are mild accounting for the difficulty in compiling accurate epidemiologic data. The incubation time is 7–12 days generally with a range of 2–30 days. Males are more commonly affected than females. Leptospirosis is considered endemic in the tropics and subtropics and affects travelers especially to these areas. Puerto Rico reports the majority of cases in the U.S. followed by Hawaii. Commonly, it is fluid borne and affects those engaging in recreational water sports and those exposed to animal urine, especially in the soil. Leptospira species infect multiple animals with rats being a common reservoir but domesticates and farm animals are also affected. Individuals who work with animals or their byproducts and urban dwellers exposed to rats are at risk. Doxycycline is an acceptable antibiotic to use, especially if rickettsial diseases are on the differential.

15.3.2 History

Exposures as delineated above should be elucidated. A bleeding diathesis is common and hemoptysis is a characteristic finding in severe disease. Other symptoms are generalized with presentations similar to viral infections. Sudden onset of fever, chills, headache, nausea, vomiting, and myalgia is common. Muscle aches may be intense affecting the calves, back, and abdomen. The headache may also be severe and localized to the frontal and retro-orbital region. Pain and headache may cause the infection to be confused with dengue initially. Reports of a rash lasting <24 h may be reported.

15.3.3 Exam

Patients may be febrile. They may have conjunctival injection that causes confusion with yellow fever and dengue (see below). They may be jaundiced like yellow fever. Other non-specific findings may be present. Examples include pharyngeal injection, generalized lymphadenopathy, and hepatosplenomegaly. A rash may be present that is either blanchable and maculopapular or hemorrhagic with petechiae and ecchymosis but generally only lasts 24 h.

15.3.4 Diagnostics

Unlike the other infections in this section, the complete blood count may be consistent with bacterial infection with leukocytosis and a left shift but only in about one third of patients. A characteristic finding is a marked elevation in serum bilirubin with modest increases in transaminases. Inflammatory markers may be elevated with thrombocytopenia which is non-specific. Renal function is almost invariably affected with positive findings on the urinalysis of leukocytes, erythrocytes, and proteinuria in mild disease and with frank renal failure in more severe presentations. Serologic tests (IgM based commercial assay) are helpful when positive but can be negative during the first week of illness. Septicemia occurs during the first 4–6 days of illness. Therefore, a PCR taken after this time may be negative and does not rule out infection. Microscopic agglutination test (MAT) is available at the CDC.

Key Points
- Returning travelers from the tropics with a history of exposure to contaminated freshwater and soil without localized findings should be tested for leptospirosis.
- The presence of hemoptysis and conjunctival suffusion together are a unique finding.
- The lab work may be typical for bacterial infections and reveals renal involvement most of the time in severe disease.

16 Fever with a Rash

16.1 *Enteric Fever*

Enteric fever is a systemic infection caused by *Salmonella typhi* or *Salmonella paratyphi*. A rash is present only 30% of the time.

16.1.1 General Considerations

Enteric fever is infrequently seen in the U.S. Rare outbreaks have been linked to contaminated foods. There are 425 cases of typhoid and 125 cases of paratyphoid fever diagnosed in the U.S. every year. However, there are an estimated 11–21 million cases worldwide. Enteric fever is mainly associated with international travel to countries with poor sanitary conditions, often to the Indian subcontinent. Infection occurs via the fecal oral route of transmission. The incubation period for typhoid is generally 6–30 days and 1–10 days for paratyphoid. Most patients with mild to moderate cases of enteric fever can be treated at home. Quinolone resistance is rising and azithromycin is a suitable alternative for uncomplicated disease. Defervescence may take several days and should not be considered treatment failure. Cases of severe enteric fever need to be monitored in the hospital as gastrointestinal (GI) bleeding and intestinal perforation can occur.

16.1.2 History

Enteric fever is somewhat of a misnomer as fever is not always present, and neither is abdominal pain, another hallmark feature of this disease. However, in severe enteric fever, elevated body temperature is almost invariable, and abdominal issues usually develop as the course of the disease progresses. In addition to fever and abdominal pain, headache (80%), and anorexia (55%) are the most common features. Other symptoms occurring with lesser frequency are chills, cough, nausea, vomiting, and diarrhea. Constipation and sore throat can also occur. Neuropsychiatric symptoms termed typhoid encephalopathy can occur. Thus, in any patient returning from international travel with a systemic illness, consideration of enteric fever should be given.

16.1.3 Exam

Fever, if present, can be quite high. A coated tongue is often reported (50%). Diffuse abdominal tenderness is typical. A rose-colored maculopapular rash with "rose" colored spots can be present on the trunk and chest (30%). Severe disease is associated with abdominal pain and is characterized by GI bleeding and intestinal perforation. Neurologic conditions such as meningitis and Guillain-Barre syndrome (see chapter "Neurologic Emergencies") can occur, as can a simple neuritis.

16.1.4 Diagnostics

The basic labs may be normal or be deranged in any pattern. Blood cultures are positive 80% of the time within the first week.

Key Points
- Enteric fever is a systemic illness associated with international travel often to the Indian subcontinent.
- Basic labs may be abnormal in any pattern.
- In severe disease, blood cultures are positive 80% of the time and are the cornerstone of diagnosis.
- Severe disease needs to be monitored in the hospital for intestinal complications.

16.2 Dengue Virus

Dengue is an arthropod-borne RNA flavivirus that has the potential to cause a fatal hemorrhagic fever which can be confused with yellow fever.

Infectious Disease

16.2.1 General Considerations

Dengue is endemic to Central and South America as well as Southeast Asia, the Pacific islands, and Africa. Dengue is the most common arboviral disease worldwide with 500,000 cases and approximately 12,000 deaths annually. Dengue is characterized by acute onset of fever 3–14 days after a bite from an infected mosquito. There are three phases: febrile, critical, and convalescent. Importantly, the critical phase begins after defervescence. Most patients recover after the critical phase with the most severe complications being febrile seizures and dehydration. However, some develop severe hemorrhagic shock. Risk factors for severe infection include infants, pregnant women, and those with a second infection.

16.2.2 History

Breakbone fever (classic Dengue) is characterized by pain such as a headache, backache, and pain in the legs. A morbilliform rash that evolves into a maculopapular eruption is often pruritic and may desquamate. Conjunctivitis, rhinosinusitis, and pharyngitis are common. A bleeding diathesis may include epistaxis, gingival bleeding, hematuria, and melena may occur. The more severe form of dengue hemorrhagic fever (DHF) begins abruptly and has associated cough dyspnea, abdominal pain, nausea, and vomiting. Bleeding causing melena and hematemesis are typical.

16.2.3 Exam

Fever and hypotension are present in DHF. Both the mild and severe forms of dengue can have lymphadenopathy; however, DHF also has circumoral pallor and cyanosis. In DHF, hepatomegaly is present and the rash is petechial not maculopapular.

16.2.4 Diagnostics

A complete blood count (CBC) can reveal thrombocytopenia. An ELISA for IgM should be positive after 8 days. IgM titers should also be drawn for Chikungunya and Zika virus.

Key Points
- Dengue hemorrhagic fever is a medical emergency since it can be fatal.
- Patients suffer from respiratory distress and abdominal pain. There is also a petechial rash. Thrombocytopenia is a typical though non-specific finding.

- The care is supportive and includes aggressive hydration and avoidance of aspirin and NSAIDS due to the tendency to aggravate bleeding in dengue infections.

16.3 Chikungunya Virus

Chikungunya is a mosquito-borne RNA togavirus that can cause debilitating polyarthralgia. Mortality is rare and occurs mainly in older individuals.

16.3.1 General Considerations

Outbreaks have been identified in Africa, Asia, Europe, the Americas, Caribbean as well as surrounding the Indian and Pacific Oceans. The incubation period is generally 3–7 days after the bite of an *Aedes aegypti* mosquito. Most patients (85%) are asymptomatic with the disease. The mortality is also low with severe disease affecting those >65 years of age and/or persons with underlying chronic medical conditions (hypertension, diabetes, and cardiovascular disease). Severe complications occur during the acute phase and cause multi-organ failure including cardiopulmonary collapse, hepatic and renal failure, and neurologic compromise. Of special concern to female patients is increased pregnancy morbidity and fetal mortality associated with chikungunya.

16.3.2 History

The fever associated with chikungunya can be high >102 °F. The initial presentation may be polyarthralgia that is bilateral, symmetric and affects smaller joints more than large joints and may be the initial presentation. The rash can be patchy or diffuse and includes the face, trunk, and limbs. Other symptoms include headache, myalgias, conjunctivitis, nausea, and vomiting. A bleeding diathesis may be present. Shortness of breath, abdominal pain, nausea, and vomiting are common. Acute symptoms resolve in 7–10 days. Rheumatologic syndromes may persist (polyarthralgia, polyarthritis, tenosynovitis) for months to years.

16.3.3 Exam

Fever should be present. An erythematous macular rash usually appears early in the infection. Joint inflammation and effusions may be present. Cranial nerve palsies can be present. Neurologic symptoms include flaccid paralysis, Guillain-Barre syndrome, myelitis, and encephalitis (see chapter "Neurologic

Emergencies"). Common ophthalmologic manifestations include conjunctivitis, uveitis, and retinitis.

16.3.4 Diagnostics

Lymphopenia, thrombocytopenia, and elevated creatinine can occur.

An ELISA for IgM should be positive after 8 days. IgM titers should also be drawn for Dengue and Zika virus.

Key Points
- Chikungunya can cause multi-organ failure with neurologic and ocular complications though the mortality rate is low.
- Symptoms and an abnormal exam of the joints are common and joint pain may be the initial symptom.
- Treatment is supportive. Obstetric complications are a concern for pregnant patients.

16.4 Zika Virus

Zika is an RNA flavivirus spread by *Aedes aegypti* that usually does not cause serious disease.

16.4.1 General Considerations

Zika virus is generally endemic in tropical and subtropical locations though infections have been reported in Texas and Florida. The incubation period is <14 days. Most (80%) of cases are completely asymptomatic. In addition to being an arbovirus, the disease is sexually transmitted. Co-infections with Dengue, Zika, and Chikungunya in the same patient are possible since the viruses circulate in the same area and are transmitted by the same mosquito. The infection is of special concern during pregnancy and to those who are trying to achieve conception as it is teratogenic like chikungunya. Rarely, Guillain-Barre syndrome, meningoencephalitis, cardiac arrhythmias, and cerebrovascular accidents (CVA) may occur.

16.4.2 History

Low grade fever may be reported. A maculopapular rash, arthralgias, and conjunctivitis may be present. Headaches and other symptoms of meningoencephalitis may be reported. Shortness of breath, palpitations, and other cardiac symptoms may be reported. Symptoms of CVA may be present.

16.4.3 Exam

Conjunctival injection may be found. Palatal petechiae may be found. The maculopapular rash is often pruritic. Cardiac (arrhythmias) and neurologic findings (meningitis and CVA) as described elsewhere (see chapter "Neurology") may be present.

16.4.4 Diagnostics

An EKG may be necessary. In patients who are suspected of Zika virus, an IgM after 8 days should be ordered for Zika in addition to dengue and chikungunya.

Key Points
- Zika is generally a mild illness which occasionally has severe cardiac and neurologic complications.
- If any concern of Zika is encountered in exposed or potentially exposed patients who are pregnant or considering pregnancy, obstetric consultation should be obtained.

16.5 Rocky Mountain Spotted Fever

Rocky Mountain Spotted Fever (RMSF) is a zoonotic infection by a rickettsial organism that can result in a severe life-threatening infection.

16.5.1 General Considerations

The RMSF is one of a number of rickettsial diseases that is endemic to the U.S. Though typically a disease of domestic travel, RMSF has also been reported in Mexico, Canada, Central and South America and may be present in travelers returning from these areas. RSMF has been reported in every state in the continental US, but 60% of cases come from five states: North Carolina, Tennessee, Oklahoma, Missouri, and Arkansas. The vector is through dog or wood ticks. Treatment should be started as soon as possible (and not based on presence of a rash or confirmatory serology) to avoid the complications which include meningoencephalitis, myocarditis, and failure of the renal and respiratory systems. Treatment is Doxycycline 100 mg twice a day for 7 days or for 3 days after symptoms subside.

16.5.2 History

Fever, headache, and myalgias can be reported with meningitis. Gastrointestinal symptoms such as anorexia, abdominal pain, nausea, vomiting, and diarrhea can be reported. A rash can be present. The typical triad of fever, rash, and history of a tick

Infectious Disease

bite is not always present as up to 50% of patients do not recall a tick bite. Additionally, the rash can be absent in 10% of patients.

16.5.3 Exam

Fever may be present. Lymphadenopathy may be present. The rash of RMSF appears 2–4 days after symptom onset and starts as a blanchable maculopapular eruption and then often becomes petechial. The rash classically begins on the ankles and wrists and then moves centripetally and spares the face. The palms and soles are characteristically affected.

16.5.4 Diagnostics

Leukopenia (despite being a bacteria) and thrombocytopenia are common abnormalities seen on the complete blood count. Hyponatremia and elevated liver enzymes support the diagnosis. These laboratory findings are common in other rickettsial diseases. Normal blood work does not exclude the diagnosis.

Key Points
- A febrile illness possibly associated with a tick bite in an endemic area could represent Rocky Mountain Spotted Fever.
- Clinical suspicion is sufficient to begin treatment.
- A petechial rash in the absence of a bleeding diathesis is very typical, found 90% of the time, and supports the diagnosis.

17 Miscellaneous Potentially Fatal Diseases

17.1 Rickettsial Diseases

Characterized by typical symptoms of acute rickettsial infections such as fever, headaches, and myalgia.

Scrub Typhus (*Orientia tsutsugamushi*) is found in south or southeast Asia in rural locations and is rare in travelers. If left untreated, scrub typhus will progress to pneumonitis, meningoencephalitis, disseminated intravascular coagulation or renal failure with fatality rates up to 17%. Two other potentially fatal rickettsial diseases are Mediterranean spotted fever (*Rickettsia conorii*) and murine typhus (*Rickettsia typhi*). Mediterranean spotted fever is found in the Mediterranean region, but also the middle east, India, and Africa. Murine typhus is found in the tropical and subtropical regions. These infections have a short incubation of 5–7 days. These infections are associated with a rash that can be maculopapular or eschar and in scrub typhus, the eschar is often found in just the moist areas of the body. Treatment for these infections is doxycycline 100 mg BID for 7 days or 24–48 h after treatment response. Failure to respond quickly implies an alternate diagnosis.

17.2 Respiratory Infections

Coronaviruses such as severe acute respiratory syndrome [SARS-CoV, SARS-Cov 2-19 (COVID-19)] and middle east respiratory syndrome (MERS-CoV) cause respiratory infections leading to ARDS. Melioidosis, caused by the bacterium *Burkholderia pseudomallei*, is a respiratory illness found in parts of southeast Asia. Melioidosis has a short incubation and can cause respiratory failure and sepsis. The chest radiograph will have upper zone infiltrates, often with cavitation.

Legionella pneumonia is an infection that deserves consideration in patient itineraries associated with cruise ships and hotels. Histoplasmosis is often found in spelunkers with pulmonary complaints, though this is often a mild, self-limited illness. TB long has a long incubation >21 days and is often seen in patients with extended stays visiting relatives in endemic areas (see above).

17.3 Viral Hemorrhagic Fevers

Patients with a fever >37.5 °C. or history of fever who have traveled within 21 days to an area where viral hemorrhagic fever is endemic or epidemic (usually rural sub-Saharan Africa) requires hospitalization and isolation precautions. Risk is dependent on exposure history, but direct contact with bodily fluids from people or animals is considered high risk. Sexual contact and funeral attendance also are considered risky activities.

Table 8 has been produced to compare the attributes of the different infections of the febrile traveler.

17.4 Measles

Measles is an infection caused by an RNA virus that causes a very contagious infection affecting mostly children.

17.4.1 General Considerations

The disease is most commonly seen in those without immunity such as the unvaccinated or infants as the low mutation rate allows for a very effective vaccine. Measles is transmitted through respiratory droplets and occasionally aerosols and

Infectious Disease

Table 8 The febrile traveler. The diseases and their characteristics

Disease	Locale	Species	Vector	Rash	Conjunctivitis	Laboratories	Special considerations
Malaria	Tropical	*Plasmodium* spp. (protozoan)	Anopheles mosquito	None	None	Decreased hgb, elevated LDH and bilirubin; low haptoglobin	Hemolytic anemia. Maybe dormant for months
Yellow fever	Tropical	RNA flavivirus	Aedes Aegypti	None, petechial if hemorrhagic	Yes	Elevated bilirubin,	Supportive treatment. Faget's sign
Dengue	Tropical	RNA flavivirus	Aedes Aegypti	Petechial	Yes	Thrombocytopenia Dengue IgM titer	Most common tropical infection. The second infection may be worse
Zika	Tropical	RNA flavivirus	Aedes Aegypti	Yes	Yes	EKG Zika IgM titer	Can be sexually transmitted, rare cardiac and neurologic complications
Chikungunya	Tropical	RNA togavirus	Aedes Aegypti	Yes	Yes	Chikungunya IgM titers	Arthritis and arthralgias severe
Murine typhus	Asia	Rickettsia typhi	Flea	Yes	No	Similar to other Rickettsial (see RMSF)	Can be acquired locally
Enteric fever	Asia, widespread	Salmonella Typhi and Paratyphi	None eggs	30% rose spots	No	Blood cultures + 80% in first week. Labs abnormal without pattern	Systemic illness, Indian subcontinent
Melioidosis	Asia	Burkholderia pseudomallei		No	No		Respiratory infection and sepsis. CXR upper lobe infiltrates
Scrub typhus	Asia	Orientia tsutsugamushi (rickettsia-like)	Mite	Eschar, or generalized rash	No	Elevations in liver enzymes and creatinine. White cells variable	80% cases July–November

(continued)

Table 8 (continued)

Disease	Locale	Species	Vector	Rash	Conjunctivitis	Laboratories	Special considerations
Rocky Mountain spotted fever	Mexico, South America, United States	Rickettsia Ricketsiae	Dog and wood ticks	90% petechial, starts maculopapular	No	Leukopenia, thrombocytopenia Hyponatremia Transaminitis	Triad of fever, rash and tick bite present only 50% of the time
Leptospirosis	International associated with water	Leptospirosis spp. (spirochete)	None, animal urine	None (<48 h)	Yes	Leukocytosis with left shift, thrombocytopenia, renal failure, UA	Aches and pains confused with Dengue
Mediterranean fever	Mediterranean, Middle east India, Africa	Rickettsia Conorii	Dog tick	Maculopapular Petechial or eschar	No	Similar to other Rickettsial infections (see RMSF)	Neurologic, cardiac, ocular and renal complications (like RMSF)

Abbreviations: *Ab* antibody, *CXR* chest X-ray, *Hgb* hemoglobin, *RMSF* Rocky Mountain spotted fever, *UA* urinalysis has an incubation period of 10–14 days. Infectivity begins before the characteristic rash and contributes to its spread. As a respiratory virus, measles is most contagious early in the infection during coughing and sneezing episodes. Much of the morbidity and mortality of measles occurs due to secondary bacterial infections. *S. pneumoniae*, *H. influenzae*, and *Staphylococcus* are common pathogens. A failure of the fever to subside after the rash is gone is suggestive of bacterial superinfection. In adults, several rare CNS complications are known to cause morbidity and mortality after the infection subsides. Post-measles encephalomyelitis, measles inclusion body encephalitis (MIBE), and subacute sclerosing panencephalitis (SSPE) arise after the infection and cause various neurologic abnormalities including seizures.

17.4.2 History

Measles occurs in outbreaks, with multiple sick contacts reported due to high infectivity. Fevers may be reported. The respiratory illness begins with cough, coryza, conjunctivitis (the 3 C's). A rash will erupt shortly thereafter (approximately 14 days after exposure). Headache, abdominal pain, nausea and vomiting, and myalgias may be reported.

17.4.3 Exam

A fever is usually present and may be quite high. The rash is maculopapular and begins on the ears and neck and spreads to the face, trunk, and limbs. The rash begins to recede after 3–4 days. Koplik spots are pathognomonic for measles and are 1 mm bluish-white spots surrounded by erythema. They appear first on the buccal mucosa around the lower molars and may spread to the entire buccal mucosa. Koplik spots appear approximately 2 days before the rash begins.

17.4.4 Diagnostics

Diagnosis is made clinically upon visualization of Koplik spots inside the oral cavity. Serology for IgM antibodies will be positive 4–5 days or more after rash onset. PCR testing of the serum is also available.

Key Points
- Measles is one of the most contagious infectious diseases.
- Patients should not be routinely referred to the ED if they are not decompensating.
- Koplik spots are pathognomonic and appear several days before the rash.
- Bacterial superinfection is common, especially pneumonia, and is suggested by fever persisting after the rash subsides.

17.5 Diphtheria

Diphtheria is an extremely rare infection affecting the pharynx and the skin.

17.5.1 General Considerations

Diphtheria is now rare in developed countries with the advent of very effective vaccination. However, immunity acquired from childhood vaccination wanes over time. Boosters are recommended to maintain protection for adults every 10 years and with each pregnancy for expectant mothers. Respiratory diphtheria is a potentially fatal form of diphtheria caused by the toxigenic *Corynebacterium diphtheriae*. Mortality associated with diphtheria is due to airway obstruction or a toxin-mediated myocarditis. Late cardiac manifestations of diphtheria are arrhythmias and cardiomyopathy. Respiratory compromise is less common in adults due to their larger airways. Treatment for diphtheria in adults is immediate administration of antibiotics (penicillin or erythromycin) and an anti-toxin obtained from the CDC. Prophylaxis should be given to all close contacts after a throat culture is obtained and vaccine administered to those whose vaccine status is unknown.

17.5.2 History

Low grade fevers may be reported. The typical history is a severe sore throat in an unvaccinated individual. Occasionally, malaise, headache, dysphagia, and voice change are the initial manifestations. Symptoms of respiratory compromise occur later and portend a poor prognosis.

17.5.3 Exam

The hallmark finding is pseudomembranes that can occur anywhere along the respiratory tract up to the medium-sized bronchi. Pseudomembranes are a thick white-gray coating that is firmly adherent to the underlying tissue unlike the soft exudate associated with other bacteria. Attempted removal of the pseudomembrane often causes bleeding. The pseudomembranes are associated with significant erythema and edema, and when they slough, they can cause airway obstruction.

17.5.4 Diagnostics

A throat culture should be obtained. Growth of *C. diphtheriae* confirms the diagnosis.

Key Points
- A patient with a severe sore throat and signs of pseudomembranes should be referred to the ED for hospitalization.
- Pseudomembranes are thick white/gray exudates that are firmly adherent and may bleed when disturbed.

17.6 Surgical Site Infection

17.6.1 General Considerations

Surgical site infections are classified as superficial incisional (involving only the skin or subcutaneous tissue), deep incisional (involving fascia and/or muscular layers), or organ or body cavity. Infections occur in approximately 2–5% of inpatient surgeries resulting in 500,000 infections every year. This estimate does not include outpatient procedures. While most wound infections will present during the period of hospitalization, the primary care provider may see surgical infections in the post-op period. Risk for infection is higher in older patients and in those who are diabetic or obese or are otherwise immunosuppressed. Other risk factors are smoking, malnutrition, cancer, and cardiovascular disease. Wound dehiscence is often an emergency most commonly encountered early in the post-operative course; however, dehiscence may occur later. In the case of abdominal surgeries, abdominal contents may become trapped in fascial defects and cause strangulation and bowel obstruction.

17.6.2 History

Fevers may be reported. Abdominal pain is reported in abdominal surgeries. Constipation may be reported with the inability to pass flatus. Drainage from the wound will most likely be reported if the wound is in the early post-operative period. This drainage will often be purulent.

17.6.3 Exam

Fever may be present. The typical findings of peritonitis with abdominal pain, guarding, rebound tenderness is seen in the case of abdominal wounds. In the case of fascial defects, a sterile Q-tip can be used to ascertain the status and depth of the wound.

17.6.4 Diagnostics

In the case of abdominal surgeries, a CT can often be used to assess the status of the wound to look for subcutaneous air, fat, and stranding, or a fluid collection.

Key Points
- Surgical wound infections are common and often need to be immediately evaluated by a surgeon to determine if suture removal and drainage is indicated.
- Wound dehiscence is an emergency.
- Incisional hernias can be complicated by strangulation of the bowel and obstruction.
- The presence of pus coming from a surgical wound should be sent to the ED if not superficially generated.

Further Reading

Aujesky D, Fine M. The pneumonia severity index: a decade after the initial derivation and validation. Clin Infect Dis. 2008;47(Suppl 3):PS133–9.

Bisno A, Dellinger P, Chambers E, Goldstein E, Gerbach S, Hirschmann J, Kaplan S, Montoya J, Stevens D, Wade J. Practice guidelines for the diagnosis and management of skin and soft tissue infections: 2014 update by the Infectious Disease Society of America. Clin Infect Dis. 2014;59(2):e10–52.

Centers for Disease Control and Prevention. CDC yellow book. Health information for international travel. New York: Oxford University Press; 2020.

Cydulka RK, Fitch MT, Joing SA, Wang VJ, Cline DM, Ma OJ, editors. Tintinalli's emergency medicine manual. 8th ed. New York: McGraw Hill; 2018.

Durack D, Lukes A, et al. New criteria for diagnosis of infective endocarditis. Am J Med. 1994;96:200–9.

Ebell M, Walsh M. Meta-analysis of calibration, discrimination and stratum-specific likelihood rations for the CRB-65 score. J Gen Intern Med. 2019;34(7):1304–13.

Guidelines for the Use of Antiretroviral Agents in Adults and Adolescents with HIV. Department of Health and Human Services; https://clinicalinfo.hiv.gov/sites/default/files/guidelines/documents/AdultandAdolescentGL.pdf. Accessed March 2022.

Havers FP, Moro PL, Hunter P, Hariri S, Bernstein H. Use of tetanus toxoid, reduced diphtheria toxoid, and acellular pertussis vaccines: updated recommendation of the advisory committee on immunization practices-United States. MMWR Morb Mortal Wkly Rep. 2019;2020:77–83. https://doi.org/10.15585/mmwr.mm6903a5.

Infectious Disease Society of America. The American Thoracic Society/Infectious Diseases Society of America/Centers for Disease Control and Prevention Clinical Practice guidelines: diagnosis of tuberculosis in adults and children. Atlanta: CDC; 2016. https://www.cdc.gov/tb/publications/guidelines/pdf/ciw778.pdf

Jensenius M, Han PV, et al. Acute and potentially life-threatening tropical diseases in western travelers—a geosentinel multicenter study, 1996-2011. Am J Trop Med Hyg. 2013;88:397–404.

Kasper DL, Fauci AS, Hauser SL, Longo DL, Jameson JL, Loscalzo J, editors. Harrison's principles of internal medicine. New York: McGraw Hill; 2018.

Liang S, Chin R. Infectious disease emergencies. In: Liang S, Chin R, editors. Emergency medicine clinics, vol 36-4. Amsterdam: Elsevier; 2018.

McClelland H, Moxon A. Early identification and treatment of sepsis. Nurs Times. 2014;110(4):22–8.

Pasternack M, Swartz M, Bennett J, Dolin R, Blaser M, Mandell D, Bennett J, editors. Infectious disease essentials "skin and soft tissue infections: cellulitis, necrotizing fasciitis, and subcutaneous tissue infections". Amsterdam: Elsevier; 2017. p. 90–2.

Rangel-Frausto M, Pittet D, et al. The natural history of the systemic inflammatory response syndrome (SIRS). A prospective study. JAMA. 1995;273(2):117–23.

Stevens DL, et al. Practice guidelines for the diagnosis and management of skin and soft tissue infections. Clin Infect Dis. 2014;59(2):e10–52.

Thwaites GE, Day NPJ. Approach to fever in the returning traveler. N Engl J Med. 2017;376:548–60.

Gastroenterology

Gregory M. Booth

1 Introduction

This chapter has been broken into two main categories of emergencies, surgical and medical, though a procedure is potentially involved in most emergent gastrointestinal (GI) conditions of both types. As the GI tract is an internal passage originating in the mouth and terminating in the anus, its various internal portions and communicating organs are vulnerable to blockage, inflammation, infection, and bleeding. As such they often need to be accessed either externally with a gastroenterologist or via a surgeon with an open procedure. The primary or urgent care clinician is on occasion the first provider who encounters a GI emergency and proper triage is necessary for a safe outcome. Proper triage is often not clear and a certain amount of experience, coupled with knowledge, is necessary to identify patients who need prompt diagnosis versus those patients who can wait a period of time until the proper treatment strategy becomes apparent.

G. M. Booth (✉)
Baltimore, MD, USA
e-mail: Boothg444@yahoo.com

2 Initial Evaluation

2.1 General Considerations

Abdominal pain is one of the most common yet challenging complaints encountered in the outpatient clinic. Acute abdominal pain can be caused by various GI disorders, but cardiovascular, pulmonary, genitourinary, and musculoskeletal disorders may also cause pain in the abdominal area. The range of GI disorders causing abdominal pain is wide with diagnoses ranging from benign functional disorders like irritable bowel syndrome (IBS) and dyspepsia to acute inflammation of an abdominal organ which may be life threatening. Some things to consider: (1) The presence of significant fever and abdominal pain alerts the clinician to a possible emergency. (2) Abdominal pain in a pre-menopausal woman without a clear diagnosis should be given a pregnancy test to rule out ectopic pregnancy. (3) In recent times, patients with an acute onset of significant abdominal pain often undergo urgent imaging, typically a CT scan, usually done in the emergency department (ED). The clinician's judgment using history and exam has to guide when an urgent CT is necessary.

2.2 History

In addition to an analysis of symptoms, some key historical items should be addressed. A history of prior surgeries should be obtained due to a subsequent risk of small bowel obstruction. Medications such as antibiotics, steroids, and NSAIDs can be important historical clues. Antibiotic use within weeks or even months can lead to *C. difficile* infection which may need immediate labs to risk stratify and guide proper treatment and disposition. NSAIDs are an important cause of GI bleeding and intestinal inflammation. Peripheral vascular disease and atrial fibrillation are often found in patients with mesenteric ischemia.

A focused history of GI symptoms can help define the clinical condition of a patient with pain in the abdominal area. The presence of fever is consistent with emergent etiologies of abdominal pain. Nausea or vomiting is concerning in the setting of acute abdominal pain that is focused in a particular area of the abdomen (see Fig. 1). However, nausea and vomiting do not always have a GI origin. Cardiovascular (ischemia, abdominal aortic aneurysm), endocrine (diabetic ketoacidosis), neurologic (central nervous system disorders and medications), renal (uremia), obstetric, psychiatric, and toxic ingestions can all cause or contribute to nausea and vomiting. The vomitus should also be described, as undigested food, bilious or feculent vomitus each define a different segment of possible obstruction of the GI tract with feculence indicative of a distal obstruction. Initial aggressive

Diffuse Abdominal Pain
Etiologies

Vascular: Aortic Dissection, Aortic Aneurysm, Mesenteric Ischemia, Sickle Cell Crisis
Intestinal: Gaststroenteritis, Intestinal Obstruction, IBS, Volvulus, Peritonitis/Bowel Rupture, Appendicitis (early)
Metabolic: Diabetic Ketoacidosis, Alcoholic Ketoacidosis, Addisonian Crisis, Uremia
Genetic: Familial Mediterranean Fever, Hereditary Angioedema, Porphyria
Miscellaneous: Pancreatitis, Narcotic Withdrawal

Focal Abdominal Pain

Herpes Zoster, Diverticulitis, and Small Bowel Obstruction (late) may be present in any quadrant

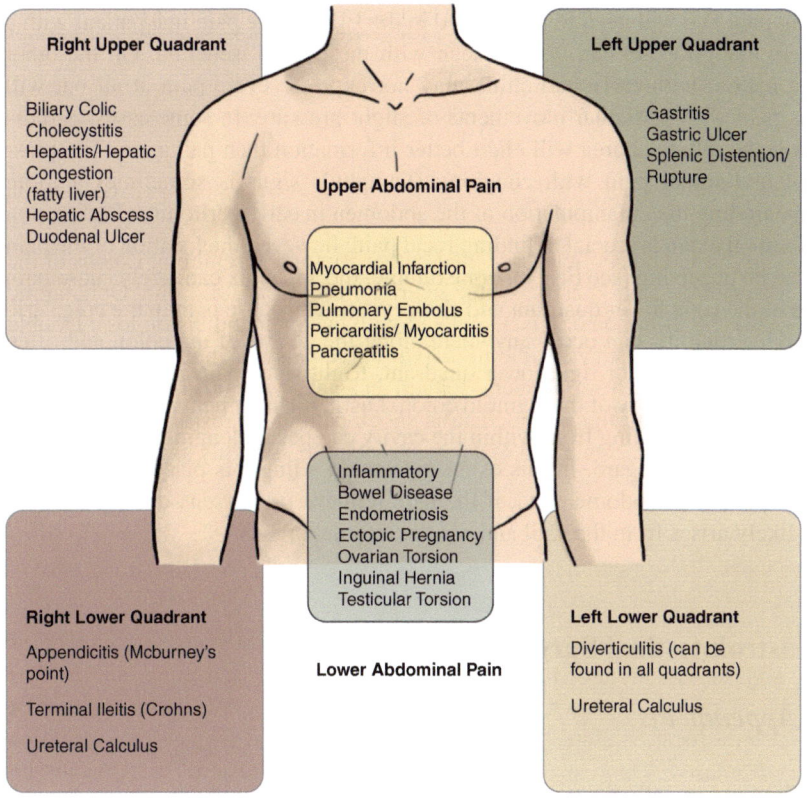

Fig. 1 Possible sources of abdominal pain by location. Abbreviation: *IBS* irritable bowel syndrome

vomiting followed by bloody emesis is consistent with a Mallory-Wiess tear which is generally benign and self-limiting. Diarrhea can also be associated with an emergency as it is found in 20% of patients with appendicitis and even more frequently in patients with diverticulitis. Small amounts of diarrhea can also be associated with obstruction or impaction as liquid stool can track around the edge of the blockage. A history of genitourinary complaints should be elicited as these can refer pain to the abdomen.

2.3 Physical Exam

The abdominal exam will also guide the practitioner which will be discussed in greater detail in the various sections below. The overall gestalt of the patient in the exam room is one of the first things the examiner will notice. A patient writhing in pain is most likely suffering the type of colicky pain not associated with an acute abdomen while a patient with peritonitis will prefer to remain still. This distinction is somewhat academic as rare conditions such as volvulus can cause excruciating, writhing pain and will need to be scanned in the ED. Severe pain in a patient with a relatively benign exam can also be seen with mesenteric ischemia. On the other hand, a patient with early peritonitis may not express severe pain at all but will express pain with particular movements or slight pressure. In some cases, percussion over the inflamed area will elicit better information than palpation. The presence of abdominal pain with coughing (Dunphy's sign) is sometimes a more sensitive finding than manipulation of the abdomen in early peritonitis. Performing an abdominal exam is crucial to finding focal pain; however, the location of the pain itself can be deceiving (see Fig. 1). For example, the appendix can rarely cause pain outside of the right lower quadrant and cholecystitis can cause pain in the epigastric region. Diverticulitis can occur anywhere along the course of the colon and often causes pain in the left or right lower quadrant. Right sided pain in diverticulitis is often due to redundancy of the sigmoid colon. Distinguishing pain in the abdominal wall from that originating from within the cavity can be challenging. Carnett's sign can be used in this regard. In this exam maneuver, a finger is placed on the most tender point on the abdomen and, if the pain remains or worsens upon sitting up, then it likely arises from the wall and not the internal organs.

3 Gastrointestinal Surgical Emergencies

3.1 Appendicitis

Appendicitis is an inflammation of the appendix, a potentially fatal condition.

3.1.1 General Considerations

Appendicitis is very common as approximately 300,000 cases arise every year in the USA and is the most common cause of an acute abdomen. Appendicitis is more common in the young but much of the morbidity occurs in the elderly population due to delays in diagnosis. When the diagnosis is unclear, laboratories should be obtained, and the patient should be followed closely. Some experts call for the immediate removal of an inflamed appendix; however, the standard of care for appendicitis is changing. Prescribing antibiotics in uncomplicated appendicitis is becoming the standard of care in some locales. However, treatment failure with this approach is common, and often appendectomy is eventually necessary.

3.1.2 History

Typically, pain begins in the periumbilical or epigastric region and eventually localizes to the right lower quadrant at McBurney's point (see below); however, this progression occurs only 50% of the time. Nausea (50%) and anorexia (extremely common) occur but usually after the pain begins. Patients may have constipation, diarrhea, or no change in bowel habits. Classically, appendicitis develops acutely over hours, but slower presentations can occur.

3.1.3 Exam

Fever may be present and is often low grade (99–100.5 °F or 37.2–38 °C). Classically the area to palpate is at McBurney's point, a third of the way from the anterior iliac spine to the umbilicus. Pain may occur in the right lower quadrant with palpation of the left lower quadrant (Rovsing's sign). Patients may have pain with extension of the right thigh (patient on stomach and right leg lifted up—Psoas sign) or with passive internal rotation of a flexed right leg in a supine patient (obturator sign). These signs are caused by irritation from the inflamed appendix. Pain in this region with coughing (Dunphy's sign) is also common with irritation of the parietal peritoneum over an inflamed appendix.

3.1.4 Diagnostics

The leukocyte count is usually but not always elevated with a differential showing increased neutrophils. An erythrocyte sedimentation rate and CRP are usually elevated. A normal leukocyte count combined with normal inflammatory markers makes appendicitis unlikely. Importantly, the urinalysis in appendicitis may indicate the presence of erythrocytes or leukocytes due to irritation of the ureter which should not confuse the diagnosis. A CT scan is now the standard of care for diagnosing appendicitis and essentially rules out appendicitis if negative.

Key Points
- Appendicitis is common and the treatment is emergent surgical evaluation.
- Subacute presentations can occur.
- In low-risk patients, outpatient blood work may be obtained and makes appendicitis unlikely if results are normal.
- Urinalysis can be positive in appendicitis.
- A normal CT scan essentially rules out the diagnosis.

3.2 Cholecystitis

Cholecystitis is an inflammation of the gallbladder.

3.2.1 General Considerations

Gallstones are present in 8% of men and 10–20% of women. Asymptomatic gallstones cause cholecystitis in about 10% of patients at 5 years (about 2% per year) and do not require surgery. Risk factors for cholecystitis are advanced age, female sex, parity, obesity, rapid weight loss or prolonged fasting. Other risk factors are family history, Asian race, chronic liver disease, and hemolysis. Biliary colic is often the precursor to cholecystitis (60–70% of the time) and shares the same risk factors and symptom complex but is separated by key differences in history. Biliary colic has a sudden onset and usually lasts 1–5 h whereas the patient with cholecystitis has constant pain. Patients with cholecystitis need to be hospitalized as bacterial infection is the etiology 50–80% of the time and sepsis can ensue.

3.2.2 History

Patients with cholecystitis typically have anorexia, nausea, and often vomiting. The right upper quadrant pain is constant and usually severe and may radiate to the interscapular area, right scapula, or left shoulder. The pain may be in the epigastric area. The constancy of the pain is the historical determinant of the transition from biliary colic to cholecystitis.

3.2.3 Physical Exam

Low grade fever may be present. Murphy's sign is characterized by increased pain or inspiratory arrest on palpation of the right upper quadrant during inspiration. An acute finding of Murphy's sign should provoke strong consideration for an ED referral. The pain in cholecystitis may be palpated in the epigastric region.

3.2.4 Diagnostic

Leukocytosis is typically but not always found. Bilirubin is elevated in 45% of patients, while 25% of patients will have elevation of liver enzymes. Ultrasound is positive in 90–95% of patients. Positive ultrasound findings include a thickened gallbladder wall, pericholecystic fluid, and sometimes sludge or a blocking stone.

Key Points
- Severe right upper quadrant pain with Murphy's sign is indicative of acute cholecystitis and should be referred to the ED.
- In patients with less severe symptoms, ultrasound can be ordered and has a sensitivity of 90–95% in acute cholecystitis.

3.3 Diverticulitis

Diverticulitis is characterized by infection of diverticula arising from the large colon, usually in the sigmoid region.

3.3.1 General Considerations

Diverticulitis usually occurs in the distal colon (95% of the time); however, diverticulitis can occur anywhere along the course of the large colon. Complications can ensue and often (75% of the time) occur on the first episode. Diverticulitis can cause perforation and peritonitis often in the elderly or immunosuppressed patients including those on steroids. Although very common and often mild, diverticulitis is still a major cause of hospitalization and has an estimated mortality of 2.5 per 100,000 per year. Liberal use of antibiotics is recommended to avoid late complications. In patients treated conservatively with oral antibiotics, a failure to improve requires admission to the hospital. Colonoscopy should be performed 6–8 weeks after a first diagnosis of diverticulitis due to the possibility of cancer as the cause of the symptom complex.

3.3.2 History

As with all abdominal infections, fevers and nausea may occur and, if present, signifies a more aggressive course of the infection. Consideration of ED referral should be made in these cases. Usually, the pain of diverticulitis is reported in the left lower quadrant; however, pain can be anywhere in the lower abdomen due to the redundancy of the sigmoid colon and is often in the right lower quadrant. Urinary symptoms may occur due to the proximity of the bladder to the sigmoid colon. Either diarrhea or constipation may be present, and there may be pain with defecation (tenesmus). The patient may report blood in the stool. The infection is often insidious and usually occurs over days, not hours, so there is time for evaluation if the diagnosis is not clear. Often the symptoms mimic that of constipation and sometimes laxatives can be ordered as a diagnostic and therapeutic tool while testing is underway.

3.3.3 Exam

The pain of diverticulitis can be palpated anywhere over the lower abdomen including the right side. A rectal exam may show heme positive stool, but false positive and negative guaiac stool is common.

3.3.4 Diagnostics

Leukocytosis can be found. Inflammatory markers such as CRP and erythrocyte sedimentation rate will usually be elevated. The CT scan is the diagnostic tool of choice and should be ordered when the diagnosis is unclear or there is no prior diagnosis of diverticulitis.

Key Points
- Diverticulitis can present with pain anywhere in the abdomen, usually in the lower quadrants.
- Strong consideration should be given for ED referral in patients with a severe presentation.
- Urinary symptoms and findings on urinalysis can be present with diverticulitis.
- In unclear cases, blood work and CT scan can be ordered as an outpatient if the patient is stable.

4 Small and Large Bowel Obstruction

Small bowel obstruction (SBO) is a blockage of the lumen of the bowel usually caused by external structures in the abdomen. Large bowel obstruction is much less common and is usually caused by an internal source of obstruction.

4.1 General Considerations

The most common causes of small bowel obstruction are extrinsic due to adhesions (from previous surgeries) and hernias (both femoral and inguinal). Hernias have a male predominance of 7:1 and are the most common surgical disease of males. Intrinsic lesions in the wall of the bowel are less common and arise from inflammatory bowel disease, neoplasms, and various iatrogenic causes both surgical and medical such as non-steroidal anti-inflammatories (NSAIDs). Congenital anomalies and foreign bodies are less common causes of SBO. Large bowel obstruction is much more unusual and is caused by large tumors, sigmoid strictures, and fecal impaction. A common feature of both small and large bowel obstruction is the continued passage of stool after the symptoms of blockage have begun due to evacuation of bowel contents distal to the obstruction. Accordingly, the presence of stool in the rectum does not preclude obstruction. Patients with partial small bowel obstruction may be able to pass flatus or have small amounts of diarrhea.

4.2 History

A history of surgeries and hernias should be sought. Small intestine blockage is characterized by colicky pain in the periumbilical or supraumbilical regions. Often the pain is poorly localized, however, focal abdominal pain can be reported. Progressive abdominal pain and inability to pass stool or flatus are subsequent symptoms. Nausea and vomiting are typical and bilious vomiting is indicative of proximal obstruction while feculent vomitus is consistent with a more distal obstruction. Pain associated with large bowel obstruction is infra-umbilical and generally less intense than that of small bowel obstruction and may progress to the lower lumbar region due to traction on the root of the mesentery. When crampy pain is followed by a constant severe pain, strangulation and ischemia should be suspected, though diagnosing strangulation on clinical grounds is difficult.

4.3 Exam

Previous scars may be present from prior surgeries. The presence of incisional, inguinal, femoral, and umbilical hernias should be sought. The most common finding is abdominal distention with or without pain. The abdomen may be tympanic to percussion. Bowel sounds may be high-pitched and tinkling in a mechanical small bowel obstruction. Later bowel sounds will be absent or diminished. The pain may be localized or generalized. Later the signs of peritonitis may be found. Rectal examination may reveal an impaction which needs to be managed in the ED with dis-impaction under anesthesia.

4.4 Diagnostics

Abdominal radiographs can usually be obtained the same day and can be diagnostic; however, CT is a more sensitive imaging modality and is the standard of care.

Key Points
- Abdominal distention with nausea and crampy abdominal pain should raise awareness for an early bowel obstruction.
- Though often readily available, abdominal X-rays are not sensitive enough to rule out obstruction and should be interpreted with caution when negative.
- A CT scan is the standard of care in evaluating an intestinal obstruction.

5 Miscellaneous

5.1 Mesenteric Ischemia

Mesenteric ischemia is a sudden loss of blood flow to the small bowel resulting in necrosis and death of the tissues.

5.1.1 General Considerations

Ischemia of the small bowel is caused by four different syndromes: (1) an embolus to the superior mesenteric artery (SMA), (2) thrombosis of the SMA, (3) a venous thrombosis, and (4) non-occlusive disease of the splanchnic vasculature. Embolic mesenteric ischemia is considered to be more likely in the older age group. The classic history is a patient who is 50 years of age or older with atrial fibrillation. The embolism causes the classic, sudden, catastrophic abdominal pain out of proportion to exam, often associated with a forced evacuation of a small amount of bloody stool. An embolic source is the etiology 50% of the time for acute mesenteric ischemia. In contrast, thrombosis of the SMA is responsible for 10% of cases of acute mesenteric ischemia and is due to atherosclerosis. The risk factors are the same as for other atherosclerotic diseases: hypertension, hyperlipidemia, diabetes, smoking, and obesity. A history of vascular disease is often present in these cases in the form of coronary artery disease, cerebral infarction, or peripheral vascular disease. The chronic disease of atherosclerosis is often preceded by a slow onset of abdominal pain termed intestinal angina, characterized by pain with eating and weight loss. The third cause is venous thromboembolism which may cause swelling and ischemia of the small bowel and have a subacute course. The risk factors for this condition are those of a hyper-coaguable state (see Chap. 1 "Cardiovascular Disease", Sect. 15). Finally, non-occlusive ischemia is responsible for intestinal ischemia 25% of the time, commonly from splanchnic vasoconstriction due to a cardiovascular event such as prolonged hypotension. This is usually a condition seen in hospitalized patients. The ischemic insult may persist after the event has resolved.

The diagnostic modality for acute mesenteric ischemia is CT angiography (CTA). Mesenteric ischemia is commonly a surgical emergency though in some cases percutaneous treatment of the obstruction can be pursued.

Key Points
- Patients with cardiovascular risk factors such as atrial fibrillation, atherosclerosis, or a hypercoagulable state are at risk for obstruction of splanchnic vasculature.
- The diagnosis is made from the outpatient setting by a CT angiogram (CTA).

Gastroenterology

5.2 Hernias

Generally benign, umbilical and inguinal hernias are palpable soft masses that increase with straining and may be associated with irritation. Generally, hernias are reducible (can be returned to their anatomic location). If the mass itself is tender and non-reducible and is associated with nausea and fever, then an ED referral is mandatory for likely incarcerated hernia. If these symptoms are intermittent, then prompt surgical referral is required.

Key Points
- With regard to umbilical and inguinal hernias, patients with a tender non-reducible mass should be sent to the ED especially when nausea and/or fever is present.

5.3 Gastric Volvulus

Gastric volvulus is a twisting of the stomach on its axis usually associated with a hiatal hernia.

5.3.1 General Considerations

Hiatal hernia is a very common and generally benign condition in which the stomach recedes into the thoracic cavity through the diaphragm. Generally, the only clinical consequence is pain from gastric reflux. However, on occasion, the stomach can become twisted forming a gastric volvulus especially with para-diaphragmatic hernias. This emergent condition is heralded by epigastric pain with retching but without vomitus. This should be referred to the ED. If the patient relates a history of epigastric pain with retching without vomiting, then a prompt CT scan of the chest should be done to evaluate the hernia as this is an indication for repair.

Key Points
- Epigastric pain with retching without vomitus should prompt an expedited CT scan of the chest, usually done in the ED. A prior history of hiatal hernia is consistent with this diagnosis.

5.4 Intestinal Volvulus and Malrotation

5.4.1 General Considerations

Intestinal volvulus is a twisting of the bowel resulting in an interruption of blood flow and necrosis of the bowel tissue. Intestinal volvulus is considered an emergency and can occur with either the small or large bowel. The most common location for volvulus is the sigmoid colon, often seen in elderly patients with a history of constipation. The symptoms are nonspecific including abdominal pain, nausea, vomiting, constipation, and bloody stool, as found in other causes of obstruction and ischemia. Though typically a surgical emergency, in select cases, colonoscopic decompression can be used to treat volvulus. A related condition is malrotation of the small intestine, a congenital condition most likely present from infancy or childhood. However, malrotation may be encountered in the adult population. In these cases, general surgery should be consulted promptly as many surgeons will correct this congenital condition immediately due to its risk for midgut volvulus. Diagnosis can be made with radiographs; however, due to their non-specificity, a CT is often necessary.

6 Gastrointestinal Medical Emergencies

6.1 Ascending Cholangitis

Ascending cholangitis is characterized by a blockage of the common bile duct and the resulting inflammation and jaundice.

6.1.1 General Considerations

The main finding of common bile duct obstruction is jaundice. The origins of jaundice can be broken down into (1) pre-hepatic jaundice, (2) hepatic jaundice, and (3) post-hepatic jaundice (obstructive). Pre-hepatic jaundice is a benign condition most commonly caused by hemolysis. Hepatic jaundice is caused by decreased uptake, metabolism, or excretion of bile. Usually, this is caused by inflammation and swelling of the liver tissue (i.e., hepatitis Sect. 6.2) which blocks normal flow of bile into the bile ducts. Another common cause is cirrhosis which affects bilirubin metabolism. Post-hepatic jaundice (or obstructive) jaundice is caused by a blockage, typically by a gallstone, in the common bile duct called choledocholithiasis (60% of the time). Other causes of obstruction are biliary and pancreatic neoplasms, parasites (especially in the migrant Asian population), postoperative causes, and primary sclerosing angiitis (PSC). Most stones in the common bile duct come from the gallbladder. As such, the risk factors for choledocholithiasis are the same as for cholecystitis (see above Sect. 3.2.1).

6.1.2 History

Pruritus can be severe and is the first manifestation of cholestasis from obstruction. Nausea, with or without vomiting, and jaundice is common with both common bile duct obstruction and cholangitis. The pain of choledocholithiasis is often midline and radiates to the back. Right upper quadrant pain may also be seen with stones of gallbladder origin. Tea colored urine due to bilirubinemia and clay-colored stools from lack of bilirubin excretion are preceding symptoms. Ascending cholangitis is a true emergency and the typical history is fever, right upper quadrant pain, and jaundice (Charcot's triad); however, this triad is found only 50–70% of the time and often not simultaneously. If a patient with Charcot's triad is left untreated, the patient may go into shock and develop mental status changes due to bacteremia (Reynolds pentad). If a condition reminiscent of Reynold's pentad is encountered in the clinic, emergency medical services should be called as this presentation needs to be addressed immediately.

6.1.3 Exam

Fever may be present and represents an emergency when in conjunction with significant pain and jaundice. Jaundice is best appreciated in the sclera (scleral icterus). Scleral icterus correlates to a bilirubin of at least 2.0. Right upper quadrant or epigastric tenderness is frequently found.

6.1.4 Diagnostics

A urinalysis in the office may show decreased or absent urobilinogen and increased production of bilirubin. Alkaline phosphatase is usually elevated in biliary disease and may be the first sign of obstruction. If an elevated alkaline phosphatase is found on laboratory investigation, prompt right upper quadrant ultrasound should be ordered. The ultrasound is not sensitive for choledocholithiasis but is very sensitive for ductal dilation of >5–7 mm. If dilation of the common bile duct is found, a prioritized referral to GI for consideration of MRCP should be performed. If a stone is found in the common bile duct on ultrasound or magnetic resonance cholangiopancreatography (MRCP), then the patient should be referred to the ED.

Key Points
- Fever and jaundice is a medical emergency and the patient should be referred promptly to the ED.
- A right upper quadrant ultrasound should be ordered for a significantly elevated alkaline phosphatase.
- The right upper quadrant ultrasound is very sensitive for dilated common bile duct dilation, and, if accompanied by symptoms or signs of obstruction, the patient should be referred to the ED.
- If an ultrasound or MRCP reveals a ductal stone, the patient should be referred to the ED.

6.2 Acute Liver Failure

6.2.1 General Considerations

Acute liver failure in a previously healthy patient is a rare condition. Various authors define acute versus subacute liver failure differently, but agreement exists that liver failure may present weeks to months after the original insult. The most common causes of liver failure in the developing world are infections, hepatitis A, B, and rarely C. In the developed world, the most common cause is drug induced, including alcohol. Alcohol mixed with therapeutic doses of acetaminophen is a common cause of liver failure. Metastatic disease to the liver, pancreas, or biliary tree can also cause hepatitis and liver failure. Other causes are acute fatty liver of pregnancy, autoimmune hepatitis, and Wilson's disease. Acute liver failure is characterized by acute elevations in liver function tests, coagulopathy, and hepatic encephalopathy. The presence of encephalopathy discriminates simple liver injury from liver failure. Hepatic encephalopathy does not always cause an altered sensorium, rather hepatic encephalopathy represents a spectrum of symptoms and signs. The more subtle symptoms of hepatic encephalopathy should be considered in the calculus for deciding the disposition of the patient. Hepatic encephalopathy in the early stages causes mood changes, irritability, disordered sleep and mild cognitive dysfunction. The second stage is noticeable lethargy and confusion. The third stage causes a sleeping but arousable state, and the fourth stage is coma. Hepatic encephalopathy can be confirmed by an EEG. Patients with liver failure should be referred to a tertiary referral center with capacity for a liver transplant.

6.2.2 History

A detailed history of drug use including alcohol should be obtained. The use of medications including acetaminophen should be elicited. Fevers, usually low grade, are associated with alcoholic and viral hepatitis. The history of infectious hepatitis consists of a myriad of vague symptoms typical for a viral illness. Weight loss, arthralgias, myalgias, cough, coryza, headache, and photophobia are common. A vague, nagging right upper quadrant pain often comes after the above symptoms. This contrasts to the more significant pain seen in obstructive jaundice. The synthetic functions of the liver become compromised in acute liver failure with the resulting coagulopathy from loss of clotting factors. (The coagulopathy in acute liver failure does not respond to vitamin K as in liver injury from obstructive causes). As a result of this coagulopathy, epistaxis, bruising, and bleeding during dental care can be reported.

6.2.3 Exam

A low grade fever may be found with infectious hepatitis or alcoholic hepatitis. Right upper quadrant pain to palpation is common. The liver may be enlarged. New onset of jaundice is the major exam finding and a referral to the ED should be considered at least for initial monitoring of the patient. Liver function may be preserved with aggressive supportive care at this junction. Jaundice accompanied by easy bruising with mental status changes are ominous signs and represent acute liver failure in a previously healthy patient.

6.2.4 Diagnostics

Urinalysis will show both an elevated urobilinogen and bilirubin. Jaundice of the skin on exam usually correlates to a bilirubin of around 4. A conjugated bilirubin above 4 should prompt consideration of ED referral. Liver enzymes are often elevated sometimes dramatically and new onset of AST/ALT elevations >400 should be considered for ED referral. The presence of hypoglycemia is a criterion for admission in liver injury. The combination of elevated bilirubin, INR > 1.5 and acutely altered mental status should prompt consideration for referral to a liver transplant center.

Key Points
- Jaundice is often a sign of significant liver failure and should prompt consideration of referral to the ED, if of acute onset.
- Jaundice combined with new onset encephalopathy and coagulopathy (INR > 1.5) should be referred to the ED, preferably at a liver transplant center.

6.3 Acute on Chronic Liver Disease

Acute on chronic liver failure is characterized by an exacerbation of chronic liver disease (cirrhosis). Exacerbations are thought to be caused by an inflammatory state, often precipitated by infection.

6.3.1 General Considerations

The most common cause of cirrhosis in industrialized nations is alcohol. A rapidly rising cause in the developed world is non-alcoholic steatosis hepatitis (NASH) usually due to obesity. Less common causes are hepatitis B and C, Wilson's disease, hemochromatosis, and primary biliary cirrhosis. The major complications of cirrhosis are variceal bleeding (see Sect. 6.5) and ascites, both due to portal hypertension. Other complications include hepatic encephalopathy (see above Sect. 6.2.1) and volume overload (ascites plus severe lower extremity edema and pleural effusions). The major issue discussed here is management of ascites in the office setting. Eighty percent of the time ascites is caused by portal hypertension, and congestive heart failure, tuberculosis, and peritoneal diseases including cancer make up the remainder. Three situations require patients with ascites to be evaluated promptly:

(1) An initial diagnosis of ascites requires analysis of the fluid via prompt paracentesis. (2) Spontaneous bacterial peritonitis (SBP) is a common complication of ascites and also requires a prompt paracentesis to diagnose and manage. SBP is defined as 300 neutrophils/mL of ascitic fluid and treatment is based on cultures of ascitic fluid and blood. (3) Ascites accompanied by new or worsening encephalopathy also requires a paracentesis. An exacerbation of ascites in a cirrhotic patient should always be accompanied by a workup—imaging and labs. (The exception is those cirrhotic patients who get regularly scheduled large volume paracentesis. Their ascites will be managed by their GI specialist). Patients undergoing peritoneal dialysis deserve special mention as they can get a similar infection to SBP with abdominal pain and fever. These patients need to be managed in the ED or in close coordination with their nephrologist. Patients with bacterial peritonitis who are on dialysis can often be treated with antibiotics diluted into their peritoneal infusates. It should be noted that patients with SBP have a high recurrence rate, 70% within the first year. These patients will need prophylaxis.

6.3.2 History

A history of drug use especially non-steroidal anti-inflammatories (NSAIDs), acetaminophen, and alcohol should be obtained. IV drug use is a risk factor for cirrhosis due to hepatitis. The diagnosis of SBP is often difficult to make as the typical symptoms of fever and abdominal pain can be absent. Often, the distension caused by the ascites is a factor in determining disposition of the patient and a cirrhotic patient with ascites can have severe distension of the abdomen called tense ascites. With tense ascites the patient may relate shortness of breath due to incursion of the ascitic fluid on the diaphragm. Ascitic fluid can also track into the pleural space causing pleural effusions furthering the dyspnea experienced by the patient—a condition called hepatic hydrothorax. Occasionally, the respiratory symptoms due to ascites require referral for prompt large volume paracentesis to relieve the discomfort and dyspnea. In patients with ascites, subtle signs of encephalopathy should be inquired of such as insomnia, irritability, and cognitive dysfunction. Onset of significant altered mental status could represent cerebral bleeding in the coagulopathic patient and a history of headaches and falls should be elicited.

6.3.3 Exam

Fever is usually but not always present with SBP (80%). A tender abdomen with ascites requires a paracentesis in the ED. A fluid wave or shifting dullness will be found with clinically apparent ascites corresponding to approximately 1.5 L in the average sized person. Shifting dullness is dullness to percussion on the lateral abdomen that becomes tympanic when the patient turns on his/her side. The distention of the abdomen can be marked in fluid overload and cause quite a bit of discomfort but usually not pain. An acutely painful abdomen to palpation accompanied by tense ascites can be caused by a thrombus in the portal vein called Budd-Chiari syndrome which requires ED referral. Absent breath sounds or crackles can be heard upon auscultation of the chest due to atelectasis and a pleural effusion (hepatic hydrothorax). Lower extremity edema of varying degrees may be found in the volume-overloaded patient. A thorough neurologic exam should be performed in any coagulopathic patient with a headache.

6.3.4 Diagnostics

In stable patients with an exacerbation of ascites, an ultrasound and complete blood count, complete metabolic panel, and PT/INR should be ordered. Based upon bilirubin and creatinine, a MELD score may be calculated and compared to previous to evaluate whether the patient should be admitted or prioritized for liver transplant.

Key Points
- New onset ascites requires a paracentesis usually performed in the ED.
- Ascites associated with hepatic encephalopathy requires a prompt paracentesis.
- Ascites associated with tenderness in the abdomen and/or fever should be evaluated in the ED.
- Significant volume overload in cirrhotic patients may need to be managed in the ED.
- When labs are ordered, a MELD score may be calculated to evaluate for prioritization of GI referral.

6.4 Pancreatitis

Pancreatitis is an acute inflammation of the pancreas.

6.4.1 General Considerations

The most common causes of pancreatitis are alcohol and cholelithiasis, accounting for over 90% of cases. However, the potential causes are many including medications and hypertriglyceridemia, usually found in hyper-lipemic familial syndromes. Idiopathic cases are common (10–20%), some of which may in fact be familial due to an unidentified syndrome. Autoimmune pancreatitis is an increasingly recognized cause of pancreatitis and can be ruled out with a negative IgG4 level. Post-ERCP pancreatitis is common and is transient and generally benign. Pancreatitis can be mild resulting in simple parenchymal edema or cause multi organ dysfunction, shock, and death. The diagnosis is generally considered to be made with two out of three of the following: (1) history and exam consistent with pancreatitis, (2) elevated lipase, and (3) CT findings compatible with pancreatitis. Therefore, the diagnosis is very difficult to confirm in the office setting as labs and imaging services are not immediately available in the typical situation. Treatment for pancreatitis is generally supportive and lactated ringers is the fluid used for resuscitation in the typical situation.

6.4.2 History

Low grade fevers may be reported. Epigastric pain is classically reported; however, pain may be in the right or left upper quadrant and radiate to the lower abdomen. The pain is unrelenting and radiating to the back 50% of the time, often accentuated when supine and relieved when sitting up. Pain usually becomes maximal at 2 h after onset. Anorexia, nausea and vomiting is typical. Patients with vomiting need to be made NPO and most will need to be sent to the ED.

6.4.3 Exam

Low grade fever may be present. Hypotension may be present in severe disease. Epigastric tenderness is most common but tenderness in the right or left upper quadrant may be elicited. In severe cases, right lower quadrant pain may be present due to tracking of contents down the right paracolic gutter. Left flank ecchymosis (Gray-Turner sign) and periumbilical ecchymosis (Cullen's signs) are rare, found 1–3% of the time (in hemorrhagic pancreatitis). Abdominal distension may be present due to ileus. Jaundice is uncommon.

6.4.4 Diagnostics

EKG should be ordered to rule out MI and pericarditis; however, ST depressions in the inferior leads may be seen in acute pancreatitis.

Key Points
- Patients suspected of pancreatitis by history and exam should be evaluated in the ED as early fluid resuscitation and bowel rest can improve outcomes.
- These patients need to be NPO and managed for pain control, control of nausea, and administration of IV fluids usually lactated ringers.

6.5 Gastrointestinal Bleeding (GI Bleed)

A GI bleed can present with bleeding anywhere along the GI tract from esophagus to the colon.

6.5.1 General Considerations

Significant GI bleeding represents an emergency. Upper GI bleeding refers to bleeding originating from above the ligament of Treitz (in the duodenum). Upper GI bleeding can be divided into variceal versus non-variceal bleeding. Variceal GI bleeding carries a particularly high morbidity and mortality and should generally be managed aggressively in the ED with input from a gastroenterologist. Established cirrhotic patients are often the victim of variceal GI bleeding; therefore, particular attention to potential liver disease is necessary in evaluating a GI bleed of unknown etiology. Other causes of upper GI bleeding are peptic ulcer disease (often asymptomatic), esophagitis/gastritis, arteriovenous malformations (AVM), and Mallory-Wiess tears. Lower GI bleeding is typically caused by diverticular disease in the colon and is painless and self-limiting. Other causes of lower GI bleeding are colitis, inflammatory bowel disease, polyps, and malignancies.

6.5.2 History

Nasopharyngeal sources can mimic hematemesis and a history of nosebleeds should be elicited. A history of drugs (NSAIDs) and alcohol should be sought. A history of IV drug use may indicate chronic liver disease. Systemic symptoms of fatigue, presyncope, and syncope may accompany acute or chronic GI bleeding. A past medical history of peptic ulcer disease may be elicited. A history of GERD symptoms (such as nausea, vomiting, bloating, epigastric burning) may be reported. Upper GI bleeding can cause hematemesis, melena, or hematochezia, or any combination thereof. Hematemesis should be referred to the ED. Melena and hematochezia should be referred to the ED if in any significant amount. Melena (dark tarry stools) represents bleeding proximal to the right colon. Ingestion of iron and bismuth can cause dark stool that may mimic melena. A significant amount of hematochezia (bright or maroon colored stool) is actually upper GI bleeding about 10% of the time, and these patients should be referred to the ED. Ingestion of beets can mimic hematochezia.

6.5.3 Exam

Orthostatic vitals (a drop of 20 points systolic or 10 points diastolic 30 s after going from a lying to a standing position) should be performed in all patients suspected of GI bleed and orthostasis represents hemodynamic instability even in the presence of "normal" blood pressures. These patients should be in a monitored setting. A good ENT exam should be performed to exclude non-GI sources of oral evacuation of blood products. Clues to a variceal source of GI bleeding are the presence of jaundice, spider angiomas, visible veins around the umbilicus (caput medusae), palmar erythema, hemorrhoids, and ascites on exam. Ascites is usually associated with abdominal distension, a fluid wave, and shifting dullness (see Sect. 6.3).

Splenomegaly may be present. A rectal exam may reveal frank blood, guaiac positive stool, or a normal examination. False positive guaiac stool testing is common.

6.5.4 Diagnostics

Hemoglobin and hematocrit may be normal early in GI bleeding. Beware of false positive Guaiac stool testing. In more stable patients who have outpatient blood work drawn, a low platelet count can be indicative of splenic sequestration resulting from the portal hypertension of cirrhosis. An elevated BUN/creatinine ratio supports the diagnosis of a GI bleed proximal to the ligament of Treitz.

Key Points
- Patients with known varices with any upper GI bleed symptoms and those with hematochezia of any significant amount should be sent immediately to the ED.
- Orthostatic hypotension represents hemodynamic instability and should be sent to the ED.

7 Miscellaneous

7.1 Esophageal Emergencies

7.1.1 Food Impaction

Impaction in the esophagus is associated with considerable morbidity and can occasionally be fatal with perforation and sepsis. The most common cause of obstruction is meat bolus impaction above a pre-existing peptic or malignant stricture, a distal mucosal stricture, or with eosinophilic esophagitis. Eosinophilic esophagitis commonly affects the young and is treated with a proton pump inhibitor (PPI) or inhaled corticosteroids. The acute development of an Inability to swallow saliva is a symptom of a complete obstruction. Other symptoms are retrosternal fullness or pain, regurgitation, or retching. Most impactions carry a risk for perforation so endoscopy is performed immediately. On occasion, a trial of glucagon is given. Complete food impaction in the esophagus requires immediate referral to the ED for a potential emergent endoscopy. Incomplete impaction may be allowed to persist for no more than 12 hours. Odynophagia or hematemesis implies potential laceration (Mallory-Weiss tear) or perforation (Boerhaave's syndrome).

7.1.2 Esophageal Perforation

Perforation is usually iatrogenic from procedures involving passage of endoscopes through the esophagus. Other causes are forceful vomiting (Boerhaave's syndrome), foreign body, infection, and tumor. Pain is generally acute, severe, and unrelenting.

The location of the pain can be variable but is focal in the chest at first and then usually becomes diffuse and found in the neck, chest, and abdomen. Alternatively, the pain may radiate to the back and shoulders and be the predominant symptom. The vital signs are usually unstable and a diagnosis requiring surgical intervention will generally not present to the outpatient setting. Radiographs show abnormalities in the mediastinal or pleural cavities 90% of the time.

7.1.3 Inflammatory Bowel Disease

General Considerations

Emergencies involving severe or fulminant colitis are generally found mostly in ulcerative colitis (UC), though Crohn's disease can also have an emergent presentation. Severe colitis in UC can be defined by the Truelove and Witts classification of UC. The components of severe colitis by this system include the historical items of >6 bowel movements a day with visible blood in the stool, accompanied by the exam findings of temperature >37.5 °C (99.5 °F) and pulse >90. Laboratories of severe colitis by this system are a hemoglobin <10 and SED rate >30. Additionally, radiographs of the abdomen showing dilatation of the colon are also concerning. Severe colitis can be the initial presentation of UC or found in a patient with an existing diagnosis. In a new patient, infectious diarrhea such *Salmonella*, *Campylobacter*, *Clostridium difficile*, *Giardia*, and *Entamoeba* should be evaluated.

Key Points
- Patients with known or suspected UC and six to ten bloody bowel movements a day, a temperature, and tachycardia should be suspected of fulminant colitis and sent to the ED.
- Hemodynamic instability denoted by either hypotension or orthostasis support this diagnosis.

8 Miscellaneous Complications of Gastrointestinal Procedures

8.1 Bariatric Surgery

8.1.1 General Considerations

A rare complication of the Roux-en-Y bypass procedure is acute gastric remnant distention. Presenting as persistent left upper quadrant pain and shoulder pain, the gastric remnant distention usually occurs in the setting of an ileus or distal mechanical obstruction. Damage to the phrenic nerve can also lead to this complication and presents as an early complication. The diagnosis is made by a chest radiograph showing a large gastric air bubble.

Early and late dumping syndrome resulting from carbohydrate load can both lead to syncope and, in the case of the late dumping syndrome, hypoglycemia. Gastric banding can cause band erosion or band slippage which is a late complication which can cause emergencies. Band slippage presents urgently with vomiting and epigastric pain and requires prompt attention. Infections of the port are usually not emergencies but require evaluation by the surgeon.

8.1.2 Endoscopic Procedures

Upper endoscopy can cause a late finding of a retropharyngeal abscess due to an occult perforation in the oropharynx at the time of endoscopy. This abscess is associated with retrosternal or back pain and fevers. Percutaneous endoscopic gastrostomy (PEG) tube placement is now a common procedure; however, complications such as necrotizing fasciitis, ileus, and tube placement into the abdominal cavity rarely occur. When placement or migration of the tube causes feed contents to be delivered to the abdominal cavity, a peritonitis can ensue. Another extremely rare complication is penetration of the bowel during insertion of the tube. This can result in feculent material to be extruded around the ostomy site. Endoscopic retrograde cholangiopancreatography (ECRP) is a therapeutic tool used in the treatment of ascending cholangitis and gallstone pancreatitis. Post-ERCP pancreatitis can occur and is diagnosed and treated as discussed above. Another complication of ERCP is gastrointestinal (GI) bleeding which occurs after a sphincterotomy. This GI bleeding can occur late, up to 2 weeks after the procedure. It is diagnosed and treated as above. Colonoscopy is a common procedure and can be complicated by a perforation which may present late. The clinical findings are that of peritonitis and are diagnosed with abdominal radiographs. A CT scan is a more sensitive imaging modality and may be necessary.

8.1.3 Medicines Used in Gastroenterology

Immunomodulators are now frequently used in gastroenterology and have various side effects. If a blood dyscrasia is found in a patient taking these medications, the patient's gastroenterologist should be contacted. Over-ingestion of magnesium containing antacids has been known to cause symptomatic hypermagnesemia especially in those with renal failure (see Chap. 5 "Nephrology" on renal emergencies). Proton pump inhibitors have also been implicated in disturbing magnesium homeostasis, resulting in hypomagnesemia which can be symptomatic.

Further Reading

Bass R, Berry S, editors. The Mont Reid surgical handbook. 4th ed. St. Louis: Mosby; 1997.

Cydulka RK, et al., editors. Tintinalli's emergency medicine manual, 8th ed. Section 6. Gastrointestinal emergencies. New York: McGraw Hill; 2018. p. 217–86.

Le CK, Nahirniak P, et al. Volvulus. Treasure Island, FL: NIH Stat Pearls; 2021.

Lynch WD, Hsu R. Ulcerative colitis. Treasure Island, FL: NIH Stat Pearls; 2021.

Tham TC, et al., editors. Gastrointestinal emergencies. 3rd ed. Chichester: WileyBlackwell; 2016.

Truelove SC, Witts LJ. Cortisone in ulcerative colitis: final report on a therapeutic trial. Br Med J. 1955;2:1041–8.

Neurology

Gregory M. Booth

1 Introduction

This chapter on neurology will have a focus on the emergencies associated with damage to the brain tissue either by ischemia, hemorrhage, or inflammation. Transient ischemic attacks (TIAs) and cerebrovascular accidents, both embolic and hemorrhagic, will be covered in detail. Traumatic brain injury and its management from the primary care setting will be discussed. Infection of the central nervous system, meningitis and encephalitis, will be briefly reviewed. Other neurologic diseases with potentially emergent presentation such as multiple sclerosis and myasthenia gravis are covered. The approach to seizures in the primary care setting will be addressed. Miscellaneous topics such as Guillain–Barre syndrome, transverse myelitis, and Wernicke's encephalopathy conclude the chapter.

G. M. Booth (✉)
Baltimore, MD, USA
e-mail: boothg444@yahoo.com

© The Author(s), under exclusive license to Springer Nature Switzerland AG 2022
G. M. Booth, S. Frattali (eds.), *Managing Emergencies in the Outpatient Setting*, https://doi.org/10.1007/978-3-031-15270-2_4

2 Transient Ischemic Attack

Transient ischemic attack (TIA) is a transient occlusion of a cranial artery resulting in temporary neurologic deficits.

2.1 General Considerations

Particular attention must be paid to TIAs, as primary care clinicians will encounter this multiple times in practice. Approximately 500,000 TIAs occur annually and 20–25% of cerebrovascular accidents (CVA) are preceded by a TIA. Proper identification and management of TIA prevents significant morbidity and mortality. Previously, the clinical distinction between TIA and CVA was time related, with TIAs resolving after minutes to several hours, and CVAs taking hours to days to resolve, if at all. A TIA, according to new guidelines, is now diagnosed solely based on the history of symptoms in the absence of ischemic changes on imaging. A TIA is a medical emergency as the average risk of stroke is 5% within 7 days and a 10–15% risk or higher within 90 days. Management can be challenging, and some clinicians feel that all with TIA-like symptoms should be evaluated in the ED. The ABCD2 criteria provide an estimated risk of stroke within 48 hours (Table 1). On a seven-point scale, 0–3 points is associated with a risk of 1%, 4–5 points is associated with a stroke risk of 4.1%, and 6–7 points is associated with a risk of 8.1%. In the ABCD2 score, 1 point is given each to (A)ge equal to or greater than 60, (B)lood pressure equal to or greater than 140/90, a (C)linical feature of speech disturbance, a (D)uration of 10–60 min and (D)iabetes. Two points are given for a (C)linical feature of unilateral weakness or a (D)uration of more than 60 min. This ABCD2 criteria can help triage those patients with possible TIA and make a shared decision in the determination of ultimate disposition.

Table 1 The ABCD2 score is formulated to calculate the subsequent risk of a stroke after a TIA

ABCD2 score		Points
Age	≥60 years	1
Blood pressure elevation	Systolic >140 mmHg and/or diastolic ≥90 mmHg	1
Clinical features	Speech disturbance without weakness	1
	Unilateral weakness	2
Duration of symptoms	10–59 min	1
	≥60 min	2
Diabetes	Type 2	1

Score	2-day risk (%)	7-day risk (%)	Risk of stroke
0–3	1.0	1.2	Low
4–5	4.1	5.9	Medium
6–7	8.1	11.7	High

Johnston, S.C., et al. *Lancet*. 2007

2.2 History

The history and exam are closely linked in the evaluation of TIA and CVA. In embolic CVAs and TIAs, intermittent symptoms indicating a TIA should be sought, such as motor weakness, sensory symptoms (i.e., numbness and tingling, especially on the unilateral face or circumoral region), and the inability to speak or understand. "Dizziness" is a special concern associated with posterior circulation TIA or CVA (ischemic central vertigo); however, it is most commonly reported with conditions other than central vertigo such as inner ear pathologies (peripheral vertigo see Chap. 8 "Otolaryngology"). Unlike peripheral vertigo, central vertigo is generally not position related and lasts longer than just several minutes. This rule is not hard and fast, as turning of the head can exacerbate central vertigo. However, in central vertigo, this effect is long-lasting, on the scale of hours, unlike the brief and intermittent episodes seen with peripheral vertigo. TIA and CVA involving the posterior circulation often evolve over 2–3 days in contrast to the sudden presentation in other CVA subtypes. Usually, a TIA or CVA of the posterior system is accompanied by other symptoms and signs besides just dizziness such as dysarthria and dysphagia and cranial nerve palsies. Very rarely, hearing can be affected in these TIAs and CVAs.

Another relatively common complaint is double vision. Painless binocular double vision can be caused by a hemorrhage or infarct in the brain stem or by potentially emergent cranial nerve palsies (see "Exam" section below under stroke). A partial loss of vision, described as a shade coming down over the eye, is called amaurosis fugax and is a form of TIA (see Chap. 12 on Ophthalmology). Visual changes can also be ischemic (see under CVA below). Seizures (see Sect. below) and migraines are sometimes confused with TIAs. In seizures, a common prodrome is the sense of epigastric rising or other auras. In migraines, patients may describe numbness or weakness beginning in one hand, gradually spreading up the arm and then spreading to the face, trunk or elsewhere, and this history is virtually diagnostic. However, migraine is a diagnosis of exclusion, and a workup for TIA is often necessary in patients without a past history of migraine.

2.3 Exam

By definition, a TIA will have no symptoms at the time of examination in the clinic. Carotid bruits should be assessed to account for possible carotid disease.

2.4 Diagnostics

An EKG should be obtained on patients with TIA though the yield is low with a normal cardiovascular examination. MRI/MRA of the brain and neck is the imaging of choice for suspected TIA. A carotid ultrasound is an option, if a TIA in the carotid distribution is suspected. Cardiac monitoring should be promptly arranged.

2.5 Therapeutics

All patients with a history of possible TIA should receive aspirin 325 mg. Clopidogrel 75 mg may be added while awaiting studies, however, this may delay surgery in carotid disease. The clopidogrel should be stopped after 3–4 weeks and the aspirin continued.

Key Points
- If a clear instance of TIA is encountered within 48 hours, it is reasonable to pursue expedited workup in the ED. This is especially true in those with a high ABCD2 score (see Table 1).
- Shared decision making may be used. If outpatient workup is pursued, aspirin and clopidogrel may be used.

3 Cerebrovascular Accident (Embolic and Hemorrhagic)

An embolic stroke or cerebrovascular accident (CVA) is caused by blockage of a cranial vessel that results in tissue damage and neurologic deficits.

3.1 General Considerations

CVAs are common; 200,000 cases are reported each year with 75% of cases being embolic. CVA in younger adult populations (20–40) is rare, but can occur due to the following unusual conditions:

- Fibromuscular dysplasia
- Cervico-vertebral dissection
- Hypercoagulable states, especially pregnancy (i.e. central venous thrombosis) and antiphospholipid syndrome
- Systemic embolization from a patent foramen ovale (paradoxical embolism)
- Posterior reversible encephalopathy syndrome (PRES) (a stroke-like syndrome with a characteristic radiographic appearance that is associated with eclampsia, post-partum, and migraines)
- Migraines (especially when oral contraceptives are used)
- Cocaine use (ischemic and hemorrhagic CVA).

From age 40 onward, the risk factors for stroke become those for other atherosclerotic processes such as hypertension, hyperlipidemia, diabetes, and smoking, and age. From 60 years old and onward, cardiac causes begin to play a role (approximately 15% of all CVA). Atrial fibrillation accounts for most of these strokes, but ventricular embolization associated with recent myocardial infarction and cardiomyopathy is also known to occur. Rare inflammatory and infectious etiologies, as seen in vasculitis and endocarditis, can be found in all ages but skew toward older populations. Although guidelines are in flux, treatment with tissue plasminogen activator (TPA) must be started within 4.5 h; however, thrombectomy can be performed up to 24 hours later.

3.2 History

TIA and CVA are closely related with only the distinction of time and tissue damage defining them (see above). While in TIA the history is paramount, the exam drives the evaluation of CVA. However, the history deserves special consideration in some stroke syndromes. The symptoms of hoarseness, difficulty swallowing, nausea with or without vomiting plus dizziness with abnormal gait are typical of a cerebellar infarct called Wallenberg's (or Lateral Medullary) syndrome. A history of trauma is usually reported for cervico-vertebral dissections. Often a car accident is the precipitating factor, but sometimes even minor, trivial stress on the neck can be the cause. Pain is often reported in the ipsilateral neck, face, or head in the case of a carotid dissection, or the back of the neck or head with a basilar artery dissection. The patient may report a sound suggestive of a bruit in the ipsilateral neck. Hoarseness can also occur due to dysfunction of the ninth cranial nerve within the carotid sheath. In cases of central vein thrombosis, a headache, which can be severe, is often reported.

3.3 Exam

A discussion of the full neurological exam is beyond the scope of this book but will be covered briefly in this section. The presence of carotid bruits should be ascertained. Horner's syndrome (miosis—decreased pupil size, ptosis, and decreased sweating) is often seen with carotid dissections. Close examination of the pupils (sometimes best accomplished in a dark room) and extraocular movements should be performed (cranial nerves 2–6). Facial findings (seventh cranial nerve) such as furling of eyebrows, puffing of the cheeks, and showing of teeth should be examined. Sudden foot drop and shoulder weakness can be a syndrome of anterior cerebral artery occlusion. Facial droop is a common sign of stroke and should always be investigated. Occlusion of the middle cerebral artery can elicit various syndromes, and focal weakness can be found in the upper or lower extremity on one side. If a patient cannot stand upright with feet close together and eyes open, this is a possible posterior CVA, especially in the absence of a clinical picture of severe peripheral vertigo. The HINTS exam (head impulse test, nystagmus, and test of skew) can be used to differentiate peripheral from central vertigo. Sudden altered mental status and inability to look up with bilateral ptosis is caused by an embolus to the basilar artery. Several visual syndromes are also associated with

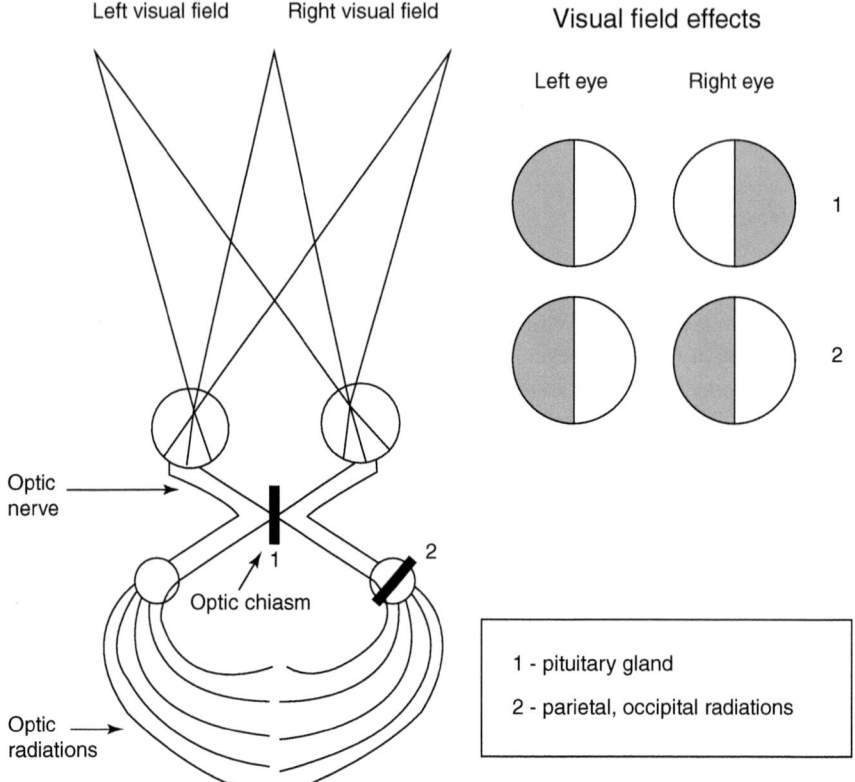

Fig. 1 1. Bitemporal hemianopsia. Bitemporal hemianopsia is usually caused by a lesion of the pituitary at the optic chiasm 2. Homonymous hemianopsia. Homonymous hemianopsia is caused by an occlusion or disruption in the parieto occipital radiations

CVA. Bitemporal hemianopsia (see Fig. 1) is associated with pituitary hemorrhage and apoplexy (see Chap. 10 on Endocrinology). Homonymous hemianopsia (see Fig. 1) can be associated with vascular disease in the parietal or occipital lobes; sometimes this finding is acute and noticed by the patient, depending on where the lesion is located.

Binocular diplopia, confirmed by absence of double vision with each eye covered sequentially, should prompt consideration of referral to the ED if acute. The exception is an incomplete third nerve palsy (sparing the pupil), almost always associated with diabetic patients. This benign diabetic cranial mononeuropathy is associated with pain one-half of the time.

Key Points
- In patients without obvious peripheral vertigo and who have trouble standing with feet together and eyes open, vertebral basilar stroke or other emergency is a strong consideration.

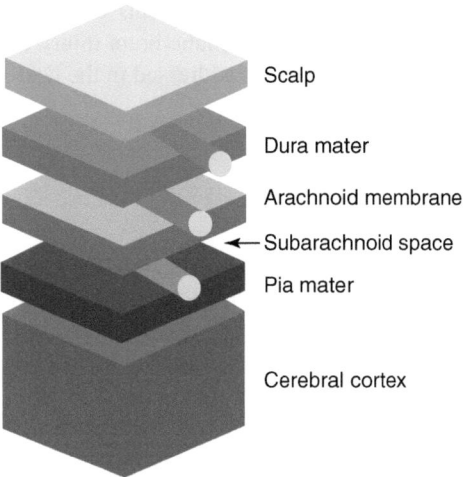

Fig. 2 Layers of the meninges

- Painless binocular double vision is usually an emergency unless explained by an incomplete third nerve palsy (see above), myasthenia gravis, or multiple sclerosis (see below).

3.3.1 Hemorrhagic Cerebrovascular Accident

A hemorrhagic cerebrovascular accident (CVA) causes neurological deficits, usually focal, by bleeding within the central nervous system (CNS). Hemorrhagic CVAs may be intracerebral (ICH), subarachnoid (SAH), subdural (SDH), or epidural (see Fig. 2).

3.4 General Considerations

Hemorrhagic CVA accounts for approximately 25% of the 200,000 CVAs that occur each year. Use of anticoagulants and, to a lesser degree, antiplatelet agents, is a risk factor for hemorrhagic CVA. Usually, but not always, the patient is older than the age of 35. The majority are ICH, followed by SAH and then SDH. A major identifiable risk factor in ICH is hypertension in addition to alcoholism. SDH and epidural hematoma is typically associated with trauma. Cancer patients can have metastatic CNS tumors (usually intracerebral) which are hemorrhagic. The neoplasms most commonly involved are melanoma, renal cancer, and lung cancer. Arteriovenous malformations (AVM) are commonly seen with SAH but also ICH and SDH. However, the most common cause of SAH is aneurysms. SAH is rare accounting for only 1% of ED visits for headache. Cocaine is often implicated in hemorrhagic stroke and patients under the age of 40 and first-time users can be affected. Trauma (traumatic brain injury or TBI) is another common cause of ICH and SDH and will be addressed in the next section (see below).

3.5 History

Family history of hemorrhagic CVA can be found, most often with SAH due to aneurysm. Patients with adult polycystic kidney disease and hemophilia are at risk for hemorrhagic CVA. Inquiries should be made concerning alcohol and cocaine use. SAH often causes a sudden loss of consciousness that may be preceded by or followed by a severe headache, thus up to 6% of syncope is caused by stroke. Thunderclap headache is a severe headache that reaches its maximal intensity in less than 10 s and should be referred to the ED immediately. "Worst headache of my life" is a historical question that can elicit a history leading to a diagnosis of SAH. Associated symptoms of nausea (with or without vomiting) and photophobia are commonly associated with hemorrhagic CVA and should prompt immediate imaging. Headaches occurring during heavy exercise and sexual intercourse are common complaints in subarachnoid hemorrhage (SAH), but SAH symptoms can also occur at rest. A headache associated with altered mental status could be a hemorrhage and should be sent to the ED. Headaches associated with sudden changes in visual acuity or bilateral double vision are concerning for an emergency. If there is pain in the eye, this is generally not a neurologic condition, as the structures in the eye from the retina moving posterior are not pain sensitive. Headaches associated with paresthesias especially unilateral (does not apply to migraineur) are concerning and a stat CT should be obtained.

3.6 Exam

The neuro exam outlined above for embolic CVA also applies to hemorrhagic CVA. Some exam specifics are notable for hemorrhages and aneurysm. Cushing's sign (hypertension with bradycardia) may be present, but it is a late and unreliable finding of increased intracranial pressure. A fixed dilated pupil can be a sign of cerebral herniation and, if both pupils are affected, the brainstem may be involved. Neck stiffness (nuchal rigidity) or neck tenderness (less specific) can be seen with hemorrhagic CVA. Photophobia to pen light exam may be prominent. Complete third nerve palsy (medial eye movement disruption with dilation of the pupil) is a posterior communicating aneurysm until proven otherwise. An isolated sixth nerve palsy can be seen with increased intracranial pressure. Bitemporal hemianopsia can be seen in disruptions of the pituitary (see Fig. 1). As with embolic stroke, homonymous hemianopsia can be seen with disruption of the parietotemporal lobe or occipital lobe (see Fig. 1).

3.7 Diagnostics

A CT of the head without contrast is the diagnostic test of choice. In the case of SAH, the CT is 80% sensitive. If suspicion is high, the patient should be sent to the ED for a lumbar puncture to increase the sensitivity of the evaluation.

Key Points
- A thunderclap headache or "worst headache of my life" are descriptions of a potential emergent neurologic condition.
- Nausea, photophobia, or neck pain may be present.
- Any headache associated with loss of consciousness, altered mental status, or visual symptoms (unless migraineur) should be considered for an ED referral.

4 Traumatic Brain Injury

Traumatic brain injury (TBI) is a closed head injury resulting in damage to the cerebral cortex and incorporates the term concussion but is not synonymous with it.

4.1 General Considerations

Approximately, 1.5 million people in the U.S. suffer a TBI annually. A TBI can cause hemorrhage within any layers of the cranium (see Fig. 2). In the primary care setting, most of the presentations will be after the fact, and the clinician must discern between common sequelae following head injury that are expected, versus symptoms and signs that need or may need immediate attention. Loss of consciousness and amnesia should always be assessed but are not always present with a TBI that necessitates emergent care. Despite this caveat, the Canadian head CT rule has been developed to give guidance on which patients need an urgent or emergent head CT (see Table 2).

The Canadian Head CT rule applies to those who have lost consciousness and have amnesia that lasts less than 30 min after the event. The Canadian Head CT rule does not apply to any patients with a seizure, on blood thinners, or age less than 16 years old. The Canadian Head CT rules state that a patient with a brief loss of consciousness or amnesia (less than 30 min), and with (1) only 1 or no episodes of vomiting, (2) age less than 65 years old, (3) no signs of skull fracture (see below), and (4) a normal Glasgow coma score at 2 h, does not need an emergent head CT. A normal Glasgow score is characterized by a patient with their eyes open spontaneously, alert and oriented (normal verbal responses), and able to follow simple commands. Two other risk factors were scored as medium risk: (1) retrograde amnesia to the event of greater than 30 min and (2) a dangerous mechanism such as a fall greater than 3 feet or greater than five stairs. Medium risk factors warranted consideration of CT depending on clinical situation.

Table 2 Canadian Head CT rule for traumatic brain injury (TBI)

High risk (for neurosurgical intervention)
GCS score <15 at 2 h after injury Suspected open or depressed skull fracture Any sign of basilar skull fracture[a] Vomiting ≥2 episodes Age ≥65 years
Medium risk (for brain injury on CT)
1. Amnesia before impact ≥30 min 2. Dangerous mechanism[b] (*pedestrian, occupant ejected, fall from elevation*)

[a]Signs of basilar skull fracture
- Hemotympanum, "raccoon" eyes, CSF otorrhea/rhinorrhea, Battle's sign

[b]Dangerous mechanism
- Pedestrian struck by vehicle
- Occupant ejected from motor vehicle
- Fall from elevation ≥3 feet or 5 stairs

Rule not applicable if:
- Non-trauma cases
- GCS <13
- Age <16 years
- Coumadin or bleeding disorder
- Obvious open skull fracture

CSF cerebrospinal fluid, *GCS* Glasgow Coma Scale
Stiell, I.G., et al. *Lancet* 2001

4.2 History

The patient will report a headache. Nausea and vomiting are always cause for concern that a hemorrhage has occurred. Of note, the post-concussive syndrome is common following a head trauma and does not require imaging though the patient may be very distressed by these symptoms and their long-lasting nature. Somatic symptoms of the post-concussive syndrome are headache, sleep disturbance, vertigo, nausea, fatigue, and sensitivity to noise or light. Cognitive symptoms affecting memory and attention as well as affective symptoms such as anxiety, depression, and irritability may also occur. As disturbing to patients as these symptoms are, especially when lasting up to 3 months, (found in 80% of concussion patients) or longer (up to a year in 15% of patients), these symptoms do not require any additional emergent imaging.

4.3 Exam

Cushing's sign (hypertension with bradycardia) may be present, but is a late and unreliable finding indicating increased intracranial pressure. A fixed dilated pupil can be a sign of cerebral herniation; and, if both pupils are affected, the brainstem may be involved. Raccoon eyes, Battle's sign (retroauricular ecchymosis), and hemotympanum are signs of basilar skull fracture. Cerebrospinal fluid (CSF) leak, resulting in otorrhea or rhinorrhea, may also signal a basilar skull fracture. The rest

Neurology

of the neurologic examination is similar to that seen with CVA, as hemorrhage is the major concern with the TBI patient.

Key Points
- If the encounter is soon after the occurrence of injury and criteria are not met for a CT, ensure that the patient is able to be closely observed for 24 hours in the outpatient setting.
- Loss of consciousness or anterograde amnesia are not necessary for severe brain trauma and the clinical rules are meant to provide guidance and do not outweigh judgment.

5 Bell's Palsy

Bell's palsy is unilateral damage to the facial nerve resulting in a syndrome that is easily confused with CVA.

5.1 General Considerations

Idiopathic facial nerve palsy (or Bell's palsy) is not an emergency but presents very similar to a CVA. Approximately, 80,000 cases of Bell's palsy occur every year. The etiology of Bell's palsy is thought to be viral and patients are usually treated with antiviral medications and steroids though the evidence for this is not strong. In endemic areas, Lyme disease has also been implicated. If function of the facial nerve has not begun to recover after 4 months, the patient should be imaged and reevaluated.

5.2 History

The onset of Bell's palsy is acute usually over a day or two and causes decreased tearing, loss of taste or hearing and sagging of the face on the affected side. More than one cranial neuropathy can occur which can be confusing to the clinician and will generally require prompt imaging.

5.3 Exam

The hallmark of the exam is dysfunction of the peripheral facial nerve involving eye closing, cheek puffing, and mouth closing on one side PLUS interruption of forehead wrinkling. (A unilateral central lesion usually spares the function of the forehead muscles due to the dual innervation of the forehead muscles). However, if the forehead is spared, this does not always imply a central lesion.

Key Point
- A lesion that affects the function of the peripheral facial nerve (including the action of the forehead muscles) is peripheral and does not constitute an emergency.

6 Meningitis and Encephalitis

CNS infections cause inflammation of the tissues of the CNS and are often caused by various microorganisms. These infections can be fatal.

6.1 General Considerations

CNS infections are not the only cause of meningitis as medications, vasculitis, and miscellaneous etiologies exist. However, the primary care practitioner should be aware that these are diagnoses of exclusion and vigilance for infectious causes must be maintained. Viral meningitis is common with enteroviral meningitis alone causing 75,000 infections every year. The incidence of bacterial meningitis is less with 10–15,000 cases per year, resulting in 2000 deaths. Encephalitis is equally as rare with only 20,000 cases reported each year. Risk factors for bacterial meningitis include previous neurosurgical procedures (i.e., shunts) or skull fracture resulting in CSF leak. Bacterial meningitis can also spread contiguously from infections such as sinusitis, otitis media, and mastoiditis. Systemic risks are asplenia, sickle cell disease, post-transplant status, cancer, and HIV. Alcoholism and cirrhosis are also risk factors. Meningitis can spread to the surrounding brain tissue and cause meningoencephalitis. This is more common in the aseptic causes of meningitis caused by viruses, fungi, and other bacterial classes such as rickettsia and spirochetes, such as neurosyphilis. Neurosyphilis is seen with tertiary syphilis and requires intravenous antibiotics. Encephalitis is a diffuse infection of the brain parenchyma causing vague, generalized symptoms with insidious onset. Seizures may occur. Viral encephalitis is more common in the summer months in endemic areas for arthropod borne (arbo) viruses. Organisms such as West Nile virus, Eastern and Western Equine viruses, and St. Louis encephalitis virus are common. The treatment for encephalitis is supportive except for cases of herpes virus which can be treated with intravenous (IV) acyclovir. Immediate treatment with IV acyclovir is necessary in all encephalitis patients to prevent morbidity and mortality as assays for herpes virus take time to complete.

6.2 History

The classic signs of CNS infections such as headache, fever, neck stiffness, photophobia, nausea, and vomiting may be absent or incompletely presented, especially in the elderly who present with listlessness and other vague complaints. Altered mental status due to cerebral edema and increased intracranial pressure is often present and is more common in diffuse infections such as encephalitis. Cerebral edema in encephalitis can lead to the characteristic vague symptoms such as drowsiness, irritability, and delirium, which is often accompanied by fever. Subtle cognitive and psychiatric symptoms may also be present. In brain abscesses, onset can be subacute with the presence of subtle symptoms for up to 8 weeks. Herpes Simplex 2 meningitis associated with genital infections is generally a benign entity and is often recurrent. However, in severe cases, genital-associated HSV meningitis may need to be treated with IV instead of oral antivirals. Sexual history may prove useful as tertiary syphilis may present without a prior history of primary or secondary syphilis.

6.3 Exam

Fever may be present. Focal neurologic signs may be present and a full neuro exam should be performed. Nuchal rigidity may be present (30%) in bacterial meningitis and is best elicited with the patient lying supine and the head passively flexed. Meningeal signs such as Kernig and Brudzinski's sign may be present but are often a late finding and rare (5%). Kernig's sign is pain in the back or contraction of the hamstrings with flexing the hip and extension at the knee. Brudzinski's sign is flexion of the hips and knees with passive flexion of the head. Petechial or ecchymotic rashes on the extremities are common for meningococcal CNS infections and meningoencephalitis from Rocky Mountain Spotted Fever (see Chap. 2 on "Infectious Diseases" under "Febrile Traveler").

Key Points
- Classic symptoms and signs of meningitis are often absent.
- Bacterial meningitis usually has a rapid onset (within 48 hours).
- Viral meningitis usually has a more insidious onset, but when the two cannot be differentiated, the patient should be referred to the ED for a lumbar puncture.
- Patients suspected of encephalitis must be referred immediately to the hospital for treatment with IV acyclovir.

7 Spinal Cord Compression

Spinal cord compression usually comes from the epidural space of the spinal CNS, most commonly from malignant or infectious causes.

7.1 General Considerations

About 20,000 cases of spinal cord compression happen every year due to cancer. Despite its rarity, the clinician must maintain vigilance when dealing with back pain, as early intervention in cases of cord compression can mitigate permanent disabling injury. Malignant metastasis to the spine is of great concern in patients with a history of active or remote cancer and is most common with breast, lung, or prostate cancer. Epidural abscess is a rare condition and up to half of these infections originate from hematogenous spread of bacteria from soft tissue, urinary or respiratory tract infections. Other risk factors for abscess are immunosuppression including diabetes, IV drug abuse and recent procedures such as surgery, lumbar puncture or epidural anesthesia. Hematoma is another rare cause and awareness of this entity should be high with patients on anticoagulation. Another cause of compression to the central or peripheral nervous system of the spine includes disc disease which is common and can also necessitate urgent intervention.

7.2 History

Back pain is present in 90% of epidural metastases and 70–90% of cases of epidural abscesses. Unlike the back pain with musculoskeletal causes, there is no positional component and the patient will not likely relate an inciting mechanism. Inability to find a comfortable position is often related. Subjective fevers are an ominous sign when occurring with back pain. The development of radicular syndromes is the first symptom of cord compromise and is followed by fecal or urinary incontinence or sexual dysfunction. Motor weakness and paralysis in the lower extremities occurs in the later stages. Saddle anesthesia indicative of cauda equina syndrome can be seen and is considered an emergency.

7.3 Exam

Searching for localized tenderness over the midline spine is of great importance. Motor weakness should be sought for with heel and toe walking and squatting on one leg. Hyperreflexia and Babinski sign indicates upper motor (CNS) neuron involvement. Cauda equina syndrome findings with decreased rectal tone (sensitivity of 60–80%) and decreased perineal sensation (75% sensitivity) should be assessed.

7.4 Diagnostics

In unclear cases of epidural abscess, CBC, ESR, and CRP may be ordered in addition to an MRI of the spine which should be obtained within 24–48 hours. Leukocytosis may be absent, however inflammatory markers should be elevated but are a non-specific finding. Findings on plain films can lag by up to 2 months so MRI is the test of choice.

Key Points
- Back pain in the midline on the spinal processes is concerning for secondary back pain.
- Unexplained back pain in a patient with a history of cancer is concerning.
- Fever and back pain are ominous signs of epidural abscess.
- In unclear cases of epidural abscess inflammatory markers can be helpful as can MRI.
- Back pain associated with muscle weakness needs urgent attention.

8 Multiple Sclerosis

Multiple sclerosis (MS) is a disease of neurologic dysfunction caused by autoimmune destruction of the myelin sheath of nerves in the central nervous system (CNS).

8.1 General Considerations

MS is extremely common, affecting 350,000 people in the U.S. and is the most common cause of neurologic disability in the young. MS is twice as common in females as it is in males. MS is defined by multiple discrete synchronous lesions in the CNS, which cause a wide variety of symptoms and exam findings. By definition, there must be more than one CNS lesion and more than one exacerbation to make the diagnosis. Usually the presentation is subacute; however, sometimes the presentation is characterized by abrupt focal signs and resembles a CVA. Most MS cases are relapsing remitting (90%), but other cases are purely progressive.

8.2 History

MS can cause a wide variety of motor (35%), sensory (37%), visual (50%), and cerebellar (17%) symptoms. A pseudo-exacerbation is often caused by stress, heat, or infections and will resolve within 48 hours with rest or treatment of the bacterial infection. UTI is a very common cause of a pseudo-exacerbation. However, MS causes progressive bladder spasticity resulting in urgency and frequency resembling UTI which often makes the diagnosis difficult. Incontinence to both bowel and bladder can occur, but this is generally a late finding. Cognitive and emotional problems are common in established cases. Heat sensitivity, the appearance or worsening of symptoms on exposure to heat (often a hot shower), is present in most patients.

Vertigo may occur and is often associated with symptoms resembling lesions of the fifth or seventh cranial nerve. Optic neuritis (see Chap. 12 on "Ophthalmic Emergencies") is common and is associated with eye pain and vision loss. Double vision or blurry vision may be due to a sixth nerve palsy or internuclear ophthalmoplegia (INO) (see below). Bilateral INO in an awake patient is highly suggestive of MS. Trigeminal neuralgia is lancinating shock pain in the distribution of the trigeminal nerve and, when bilateral in a patient under 50, is highly suggestive of MS.

8.3 Exam

Lhermitte sign is classic though not entirely specific for MS and is described as electric shocks, vibration, or pain radiating down the back and often into the legs caused by flexion of the neck. It is rare at approximately 3%. Strength may be decreased in a focal or more generalized pattern. Pain and temperature sensation may be decreased. Optic neuritis with loss of central vision (see Chapter on "Ophthalmic Emergencies") is the presenting finding in 30% of MS patients. INO is characterized by failure of eye adduction and accompanying horizontal nystagmus of the abducting eye and, when bilateral, is strongly suggestive of MS. As MS is a disease of the central nervous system, hyperreflexia is present. Vertigo is accompanied by ataxia and nystagmus without latency, direction reversal, or fatigue. Hearing loss, facial hemispasm, or facial nerve palsy may occur but are rare.

8.4 Diagnostics

MRI of the brain and spine is used to identify an exacerbation.

Key Points
- Management of MS exacerbations is extremely challenging and should ideally be managed in close conjunction with the patient's neurologist.
- Monosymptomatic presentations can be managed with prompt MRI testing.
- More moderate or severe presentations are managed with IV steroids after hospitalization.
- Pseudo-exacerbations are often caused by UTI.

9 Myasthenia Gravis

Myasthenia gravis is a failure of the electrical impulse to conduct at the neuromuscular junction caused by autoantibodies to the acetylcholine receptor on the postsynaptic membrane.

9.1 General Considerations

Approximately, 90,000 cases of MG occur annually. The disease may appear alone or in conjunction with other autoimmune disorders such as Grave's disease or lupus. The peak incidence is 20–30 years old in women and 50–60 years old in men. The outpatient clinician may be diagnosing the condition or managing an exacerbation. In both situations, a myasthenic crisis may result in a sudden worsening of muscular function including the respiratory muscles resulting in the need for a monitored setting. A common precipitating factor is an infection. High dose steroids should not be used initially as this can cause a paradoxical weakening in one third of patients.

9.2 History

Exacerbations can be caused by infections, treatment with certain drugs, or occur spontaneously. Sensory symptoms and pain are absent. The cardinal pattern of MG is fluctuating motor weakness. Repeated use of a muscle results in weakening which is at least partially relieved by rest of the affected muscle(s). Double vision that improves by resting the eyes with lids closed may occur. Difficulty swallowing and speaking implies involvement of the bulbar muscles and may portend respiratory collapse.

9.3 Exam

There are many exam findings that strongly suggest MG. The presence of weakness of the face muscles occurs in 80% of patients and along with levator palpebrae weakness (ptosis) with sparing of the pupils is virtually diagnostic. This differentiates MG from botulism where the pupils are affected. The effect on the facial muscles causes the characteristic "snarl" when the patient is asked to smile. Counting backward from 100 may cause the speech to become slurred and indistinct. A finding that is improved with rest. Sustained gaze in one direction may worsen double vision and can be corrected by resting the eyes. The skeletal muscles may be affected in virtually any pattern with proximal muscles usually more affected than distal muscles. Reflexes are usually intact unless the weakness is severe.

Key Points
- MG should be considered in the differential in any case of muscle weakness.
- The pupils are unaffected by MG.
- Exacerbations can be caused by infections and common drugs including statins, steroids, and antibiotics.

- MG can cause sudden severe weakness of the muscles and these patients should usually be hospitalized. This is especially true when muscles of the pharynx are compromised as this is commonly associated with respiratory compromise.

10 Seizures

Seizure is abnormal discharging of neurons that can occur in various locations in the brain resulting in partial or generalized sensory, motor, autonomic, or psychic symptoms.

10.1 General Considerations

The primary care physician does not need to know the details on how to manage an acute seizure. But occasionally, a patient will present to the provider after the event, with or without a clear diagnosis. For safety, the patient should be told that they cannot drive. Some states require that the clinician report the patient to the Department of Motor Vehicles (DMV). Driving is less of an issue with epileptic patients, and they should be referred back to their neurologists after ordering blood levels of their anticonvulsants, if necessary. A seizure that is idiopathic is referred to as a primary seizure. Otherwise, seizures are referred to as secondary and have a variety of causes such as active CVA, CNS infections (such as HIV), hypoglycemia (very common), and electrolyte abnormalities. Overdoses (alcohol, cocaine, and tricyclic antidepressants) and eclampsia are also precipitants of secondary seizures.

10.2 History

A seizure often has various auras, especially a sense of epigastric rising. Various automatisms such as lip smacking, swallowing, chewing, or fumbling may be described. Behavioral symptoms may be seen, and non-convulsive status epilepticus (NCS) may be responsible for non-resolving psychiatric symptoms following primary or secondary seizures. The patient may report unilateral motor symptoms following the seizure, termed Todd's paralysis, often the sign of a structural brain lesion. Incontinence and biting along the lateral surfaces of the tongue (as opposed to the tip of the tongue seen in syncope) are classically reported. Hypoglycemia is a common cause for seizures, and other symptoms of hypoglycemia should be ascertained (such as faintness, tremor, nausea, or diaphoresis). Unfortunately, these symptoms can be confused with vasovagal syncope. Additionally, syncope can cause convulsions, a condition termed convulsive syncope (see Chap. 1 on "Syncope in Cardiovascular Disease"). The convulsions in seizure usually are more dramatic and longer lasting approximately 2 min or more. Syncope and seizure are difficult to diagnose on clinical grounds and often specialists in both the fields of neurology and cardiology will need to be consulted.

10.3 Exam

The primary care physician will encounter a normal physical exam by the time the patient presents to the office. However, NCS should be on the differential of behavior changes after the seizure event.

10.4 Diagnostics

A finger stick can be performed in the office that may signal hypoglycemia as the cause for the seizure.

Key Points
- If hypoglycemia can be identified as the cause for a secondary seizure, then a workup can be obtained as an outpatient. Otherwise, a referral to the ED for expedited workup of a first seizure (CT and labs) should be considered if outpatient studies cannot be obtained quickly.
- Non-convulsive status epilepticus may be responsible for behavioral changes after a seizure.

11 Miscellaneous

11.1 Guillain–Barre Syndrome

Guillain–Barre syndrome (GBS) is an acute polyneuropathy caused by inflammation of the myelin sheath of peripheral nerves by an autoimmune mechanism.

11.2 General Considerations

GBS is rare with approximately 3500 cases annually in the U.S. This autoimmune reaction is associated with various infections classically *Campylobacter jejuni* or vaccinations which is an extremely rare event. Other associations are the herpes class of viruses (EBV, CMV) and surgical procedures. Protein in the CSF becomes elevated by the first week of symptoms. A normal lumbar puncture does not rule out the diagnosis because protein can be absent at the beginning of symptoms. The treatment is intravenous immunoglobulin (IVIG) or plasmapheresis.

11.3 History

A preceding illness can be identified approximately one-third of the time, often gastrointestinal or viral. Often the first report is difficulty getting out of a car or standing from a seated position. Difficulty climbing stairs is sometimes the first report. Aching pain may be present in the thighs and back. This is followed by a gradual onset of weakness (days to weeks) usually in an ascending pattern from legs upward. Sometimes the weakness can have an explosive onset and happen within a day or two. The cranial nerves can be affected. In the Fisher variant, the weakness begins in the face and upper body first, sometimes with ataxia, and can be confused with myasthenia gravis or CVA. Sensory symptoms are lacking or mild and are not noticed because pain fibers are not generally involved. Autonomic dysfunction may be present, resulting in difficulty urinating or constipation. Facial flushing may be reported. Presyncope may be reported due to orthostatic blood pressures. The diaphragm may be affected causing a gradual onset of shortness of breath.

11.4 Exam

Blood pressure may be high or low depending on the position of the patient. Autonomic dysfunction is differentiated from orthostasis by being sustained more than 30 seconds. Due to autonomic dysfunction, the heart rate may be fluctuating with tachycardia or bradycardia. An ophthalmoplegia or other cranial neuropathies, especially the facial nerve, may be present (50% of the time) and usually will be bilateral. The weakness is usually symmetrical and will typically be ascending found in the lower extremities first. Hyporeflexia or areflexia will be elicited due to the peripheral nature of this nervous system disorder.

Key Points
- GBS is a rare peripheral neuropathy causing paralysis, usually in an ascending pattern, and autonomic dysfunction.
- Cranial nerves especially the facial nerve can be affected.
- GBS can cause respiratory compromise and the patient needs to be in a monitored setting.

12 Transverse Myelitis

Transverse myelitis is an inflammation of the spinal cord causing neurologic deficits downstream of the lesion.

12.1 General Considerations

The condition is rare with approximately 1500 cases reported annually in the U.S. Up to 40% of cases are associated with an antecedent infection. Many infections have been associated such as influenza, herpes viruses (EBV and CMV), the childhood viruses (measles, mumps, and rubella), and varicella. Multiple sclerosis may also be implicated in some cases.

12.2 History

The initial symptom is focal neck or back pain followed by various combinations of sensory symptoms, weakness, and sphincter dysfunction. Urinary retention or overflow incontinence can be reported. Isolated hemicord involvement can cause unilateral symptoms. The symptoms can evolve quickly within hours or develop within days. The symptoms can start distally and ascend like Guillain–Barre syndrome (GBS); however, involvement of the trunk is the distinction between the two entities.

12.3 Exam

A sharply demarcated cord level is seen on sensory exam. Weakness in the arms and/or legs is typical. Hyperreflexia is the rule but areflexia can be seen with spinal shock.

Key Points
- Transverse myelitis is an emergency characterized by a sensory cord level on the trunk.
- The treatment is IV steroids after hospitalization.

13 Wernicke's Encephalopathy

Wernicke's encephalopathy is a constellation of neurologic symptoms caused by deficiency of thiamine (vitamin B1).

13.1 General Considerations

This is mainly a disease of alcoholics though only a fraction of alcoholics develop these symptoms. Wernicke disease is also associated with malnutrition, renal dialysis, cancer or acquired immune deficiency syndrome (AIDS).

13.2 History

A history of disorders of malnutrition should be obtained. A history of alcoholism may be related as well. Double vision and difficulty ambulating may be reported. In many instances, the patient will be confused or indifferent and inattentive.

13.3 Exam

Ophthalmoplegia is characterized by lateral rectus palsy (usually bilateral) and horizontal nystagmus on lateral gaze. Ptosis and miosis may rarely occur. A wide based gait with inability to tandem walk is observed.

Key Points
- Wernicke's disease is a medical emergency as lack of IV thiamine can result in stupor and death.
- A patient who is suspected to have Wernicke's encephalopathy should be referred to the ED.

14 Botulism

Botulism is an extremely rare, life-threatening neuromuscular disease caused by the bacterium *Clostridium botulinum*.

14.1 General Considerations

Botulism is covered in the neurology section due to its dramatic neurologic sequelae. Botulism is toxin mediated and adults can acquire the condition via infected food or an infected wound. The disease is extremely rare with only reports of roughly 23 cases of food borne botulism per year. Food borne botulism is associated with a low pH, low salt, low sugar environment often seen with home canning. Wound botulism is often associated with injection drug users, especially black tar heroin tissue injection. The disease progresses throughout the entire body eventually affecting all the skeletal muscles including the diaphragm. The result is asphyxiation and death.

14.2 History

A history of home canning or injection drug use may be reported. In foodborne botulism, abdominal pain, nausea, and vomiting may be reported 12–72 h after food ingestion. Double vision is reported. Dysphagia, dysphonia, and slurred speech are common termed bulbar symptoms. Altered mental status is not reported as the toxin does not cross the blood–brain barrier.

14.3 Exam

Multiple cranial nerves are affected therefore isolated palsies are often not seen. Cranial nerve palsies are symmetrical causing bilateral ptosis and bilateral pupillary dilation. The patient may be slurring words. Weakness of muscles can be reported in any combination throughout the body.

Key Points
- Botulism is an extremely rare toxin mediated condition characterized by multiple symmetrical cranial nerve palsies with dilation of the pupils. The toxin can be generated by clostridium found in canned goods or infected wounds.
- The diagnosis is clinical, and the Centers for Disease Control and Prevention (CDC) has a 24-h hotline for consultations in suspected cases.

Further Reading

Amarenco P, et al. Transient ischemic attack. N Engl J Med. 2020;382:1933–41.

Cydulka RK, Fitch MT, Joing SA, Wang VJ, Cline DM, Ma OJ, editors. Tintinalli's emergency medicine manual. 8th ed. New York: McGraw Hill; 2018.

https://www.uptodate.com/contents/initial-evaluation-and-management-of-transient-ischemic-attack-and-minor-ischemic-stroke. Accessed 16 Feb 2021.

Iain AJ, Shahnawaz K. Botulism. Treasure Island (FL): StatPearls Publishing; 2021.

Jameson JL, Fauci AS, Kasper DL, Hauser SL, Longo DL, Loscalzo J, editors. Harrison's principles of internal medicine. 20th ed. New York: McGraw Hill; 2018.

Johnston SC, Rothwell PM, Nguyen-Huynh MN, et al. Validation and refinement of scores to predict very early stroke risk after transient ischeamic attack. Lancet. 2007;369(9558):283–92.

Stiell IG, et al. The Canadian CT head rule for patients with minor head injury. Lancet. 2001;357:1391–6.

Silva GT, Bergmann A, Thuler LC. Incidence, associated factors, and survival in metastatic spinal cord compression secondary to lung cancer. Spine J. 2015;15(6):1263–9.

Tenny S, Thorrell W. Intracranial hemorrhage. Treasure Island (FL): StatPearls Publishing; 2021.

Nephrology

Gregory M. Booth

1 Introduction

The kidney's function relies on two main structures: the glomeruli which filters blood and the tubules and collecting ducts which remove filtered waste products, maintain fluid balance, and maintain electrolyte equilibrium (Fig. 1). This chapter will focus on acute renal failure (ARF) that is commonly referred to as acute kidney injury (AKI). AKI is subdivided according to etiology as pre-renal, intrinsic, and post-renal. AKI, if left untreated, can lead to irreparable renal failure and severe consequences. Much of AKI is asymptomatic and occurs in hospitalized patients, but occasionally an elevated creatinine level will be encountered in lab work ordered from the primary care setting that requires urgent attention. Thus, in the primary care setting, the diagnosis of AKI is often made post hoc, and the decision to hospitalize for AKI is made based on parameters that will be discussed in this chapter. Following the discussion on AKI, the chapter will have brief discussions of the various electrolyte abnormalities commonly seen in clinical practice and their management.

G. M. Booth (✉)
Baltimore, MD, USA
e-mail: boothg444@yahoo.com

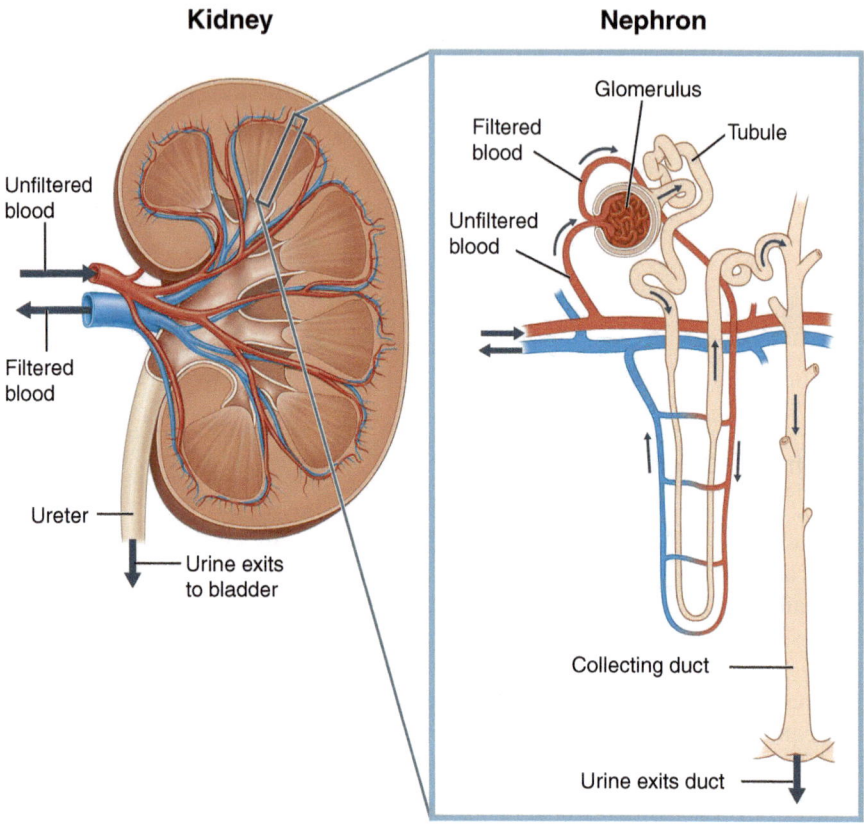

Fig. 1 Anatomy of the kidney. (Image credit: National Institute of Diabetes and Digestive and Kidney Diseases. National Institutes of Health)

2 Acute Kidney Injury

2.1 General Considerations

In general, new-onset renal failure requires hospital admission in the absence of a new drug or clearly reversible pre-renal etiology (see below). The etiology of AKI is broken down into three categories: pre-renal, intrinsic, and post-renal. In pre-renal dysfunction, the kidneys themselves are normal and extrinsic pathophysiology in the flow of blood to the kidney is causative. Intrinsic AKI is characterized by intra-renal damage. In post-renal AKI, dysfunction occurs in the drainage and storage of urine.

For purposes of the outpatient setting, AKI is strictly defined by an increase in serum creatinine of greater than 50% within 1 week or a noticeable reduction in urine volume. This definition can create difficulty when interpreting a creatinine value with no recent baseline, so close follow-up is often necessary when pursuing outpatient monitoring. Assigning exact values to an increase of creatinine requiring ED referral is difficult and depends on the clinical scenario and the patient's baseline (if available). It should be noted that at lower values of creatinine, a relatively small increase over baseline creatinine implies a significant decrease in glomerular filtration rate (GFR), a more accurate calculation of kidney function (see Fig. 2).

Uremia is the term for the toxicity related to renal failure, and its symptoms and signs occur insidiously. Although the blood urea nitrogen (BUN) is used as a surrogate for uremia, it does not correlate exactly with the severity of uremia as there is a variety of unmeasured toxins in the uremic syndrome. With this in mind, a BUN of over 100 is often considered a threshold for dialysis regardless of the severity of patient symptoms. The pericarditis or uremic frost of uremia is rarely seen but are clear signs for admission.

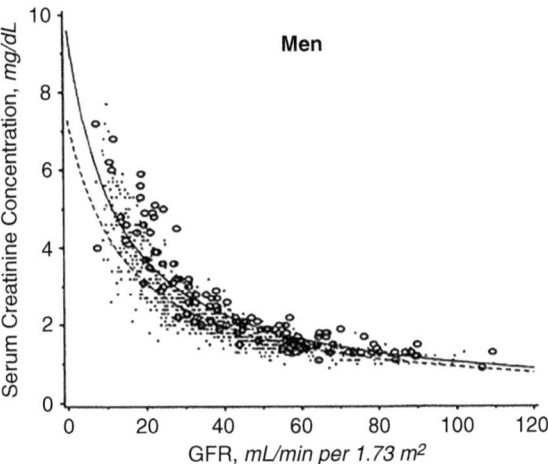

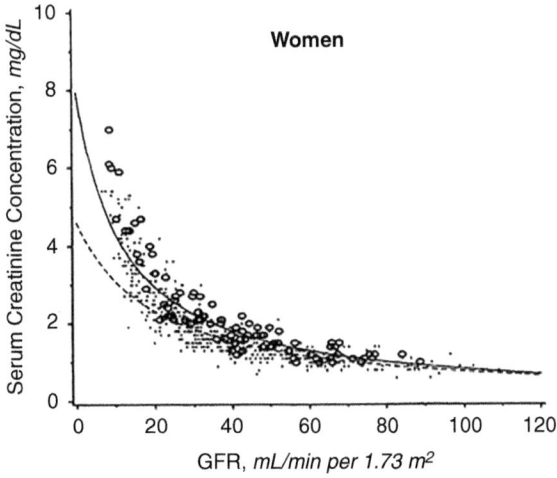

Fig. 2 Relationship of serum creatinine to measured glomerular filtration rate (GFR) in the Modification of Diet in Renal Disease Study. Note that small increases in serum creatinine cause dramatic decreases in the GFR. (Levey et al. *Ann Intern Med* 1999)

2.2 History

Severe uremia occurs insidiously with fatigue, weakness, somnolence, cognitive dysfunction, and nausea the common symptoms. Pruritus and restless legs are other symptoms. An unpleasant metallic taste may be present in the mouth. Muscle cramps and paresthesias may be present due to severe hypocalcemia. Palpitations from arrythmias due to hyperkalemia may also be a presenting symptom.

2.3 Exam

Asterixis, a flapping of extended wrists, can be present with profound uremia. Uremic fetor, a urine smell of the patient's breath, is caused by ammonia products in the blood. Myoclonus may be present due to electrolyte disarray. The patient must be hospitalized if a pericardial friction rub is heard with the symptoms of uremia.

2.4 Diagnostics

The metabolic panel may show electrolyte disarray when the GFR is extremely decreased. Hyperkalemia and hypocalcemia are prominent findings. The EKG may be normal in uremic pericarditis. Peaked T-waves may be an early EKG finding in patients with hyperkalemia. Prolonged QT may be seen in patients with severe hypocalcemia (see Fig. 3 for an EKG of a patient with renal failure).

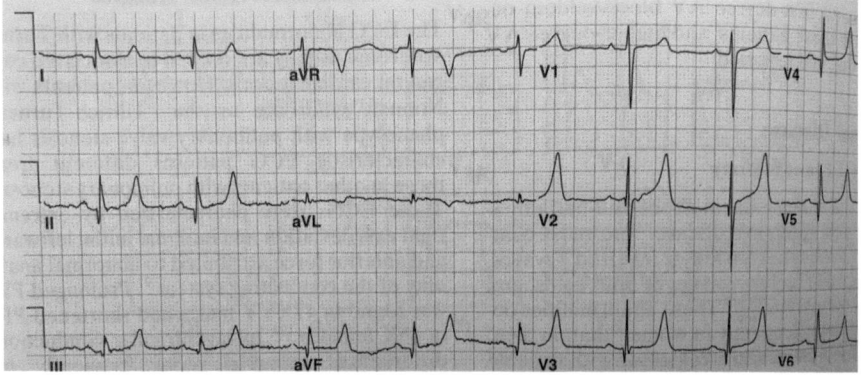

Fig. 3 An EKG of a patient in acute renal failure. Note the peaked T-waves of hyperkalemia in the lateral leads and the prolonged QT from hypocalcemia. The potassium was 6.2 and the calcium was 3.3. (From Surawicz and Knilans *Chou's Electrocardiography in Clinical Practice.* 2001. Used with permission)

Key Points
- Symptomatic uremia or BUN of greater than 100 is generally an indication for dialysis.
- Uremia is often accompanied by significant electrolyte disarray.
- Pericarditis encountered in a setting of uremia needs management in the hospital.
- EKGs in uremic patients with pericarditis are often normal.

3 Pre-renal Acute Kidney Injury

3.1 General Considerations

Pre-renal AKI is by far the most common form of AKI, accounting for about 70% of community acquired AKI. Pre-renal AKI is usually caused by a lack of blood flow to the kidney. Hypotension from fluid loss or other clinical scenarios, such as those found in heart failure or cirrhosis, are often the reason for ED referral. Non-steroidal anti-inflammatory drugs (NSAIDs), especially when combined with ACE inhibitors, are another common cause of pre-renal AKI. Pre-renal AKI can progress to a more subacute condition through ischemic damage of the tubules called acute tubular necrosis (ATN). Most of the time, a significant increase in creatinine from baseline is necessary to raise concern in pre-renal AKI. A notable exception is the relatively minor change in serum creatinine that requires hospitalization in some cirrhotic patients with hepatorenal syndrome. As creatinine is a breakdown product of skeletal muscle, the patient's weight and amount of muscle mass plays a role in evaluating creatinine levels in cachectic patients with cirrhosis.

3.2 History

Various causes of hypotension are responsible for pre-renal AKI. Symptoms related to volume loss are often present. Examples are vomiting or diarrhea. A history of recent initiation of NSAIDs or ACE inhibitors or angiotensin receptor blockers (ARBs) is common. Symptoms of anemia may be present with AKI and a hemoglobin less than 7 requires transfusion (see Chap. 11 on "Hematology/Oncology").

3.3 Exam

Hypotension or orthostasis is often present. Decreased skin turgor or dry mucous membranes may be present with hypovolemic causes of pre-renal AKI. Neck veins may be flat. Heart failure (see Chap. 1 on "Cardiovascular Disease") or cirrhosis (see Chap. 3 on "Gastroenterology") can cause pre-renal AKI and the examination findings of these disorders can be found.

3.4 Diagnostics

The laboratory evaluation of AKI includes a CBC, basic metabolic panel, and urinalysis with microscopy. In pre-renal AKI, the urinalysis is often normal or contains hyaline casts. Anemia may or may not be present. A renal ultrasound can distinguish between chronic (scarring and atrophy) disease versus acute injury (normal or edema).

Key Points
- Pre-renal disease in otherwise healthy patients often responds to fluid intake (either IV or oral depending on the clinical scenario).
- Worsening hepatorenal syndrome can be associated with relatively minor increases in the serum creatinine of cachectic patients and requires hospitalization.

4 Intrinsic Renal Disease

4.1 General Considerations

A full discussion of intrinsic renal disease is beyond the scope of this book and the information below is both general and incomplete. However, broadly speaking, intrinsic renal disease affects either the glomeruli or the tubulointerstitial system (see Fig. 1) and is a relatively rare cause of AKI (5%). Intrinsic renal disease that requires admission usually is part of a systemic condition. An example is nephritic glomerulonephritis which has typical physical and laboratory findings: hypertension, edema, hematuria (usually microscopic), and proteinuria. Diseases of the renal interstitium and renal tubules are another cause of AKI and have a variety of causes including drugs such as antibiotics, NSAIDs, infections, and autoimmune disorders (lupus, Sjogren's). A rising cause of tubulointerstitial disease is the novel medications used in oncology such as tyrosine kinase inhibitors (See Table 1). Allergic interstitial nephritis (AIN) is a condition caused by an offending agent and can have a rapidly progressive course. The classic presentation of AIN (arthralgias, a fever, rash, peripheral and urinary eosinophilia after a b-lactam antibiotic) is rare, and this entity must be suspected with any initiation of a new medication and AKI. Another rare cause of intrinsic renal disease is inflammation (vasculitis) or compromise of the renal microcirculation. Several forms of vasculitis (ANCA vasculitides) and the pulmonary-renal disease of Goodpasture's syndrome are also causative. Vasculitis and Goodpasture's syndrome generally require ED referral.

Microangiopathic hemolytic anemia (MAHA) is a form of thrombotic microangiopathy characterized by thrombocytopenia and renal failure (see Table 1). Most forms of thrombotic microangiopathy (TMA) are associated with MAHA. MAHA can be drug-induced and some anti-cancer drugs such as gemcitabine, VEGF-inhibitors, and proteasome inhibitors are culprits.

Table 1 Does not represent a complete list of disorders causing intrinsic renal disease

Nephritic glomerulonephritis	Interstitial nephritis	Vascular injury

Post-streptococcal glomerulonephritis
Lupus nephritis
IgA nephropathy (rare)
ANCA small vessel vasculitis
Granulomatosis with polyangiitis (Wegener's)
Microscopic polyangiitis
Churg's Strauss
Henoch–Schonlein purpura
Hepatitis C (cryoglobulinemia)
	Medications
	  Antibiotics especially B-Lactams
	  NSAIDS
	  PPIs, H2 blockers
	  Allopurinol
	  Diuretics
	Infections
	  Bacteria-strep., staph, and legionella
	  Viruses—EBV, CMV, HIV
	Autoimmune
	  Sjogren's
	  Lupus
	Obstructive
	  Myeloma
	  Urate nephropathy
		Hypertensive nephropathy
		Antiphospholipid syndrome
		MAHA
		Thrombotic thrombocytopenia Purpura (TTP)
		Hemolytic uremic syndrome (HUS)
		Scleroderma renal crisis (50%)
		HELLP syndrome (similar to MAHA)
		HIV TMA nephropathy
		Sickle cell nephropathy

This table outlines common causes of glomerular, interstitial, and vascular disorders of the kidney

ANCA anti-neutrophil cytoplasmic antibodies, *CMV* cytomegalovirus, *EBV* Epstein–Barr virus, *HELLP* hemolysis, elevated liver enzymes, and low platelets, *MAHA* microangiopathic hemolytic anemia, *NSAIDS* non-steroidal anti-inflammatory drugs, *PPI* proton pump inhibitors, *TMA* thrombotic microangiopathy

4.2 History

The patient may have a previous history of HIV, hepatitis C, lupus, and Sjogren's disease (see Table 1). Initiation of a new drug may be reported (see Table 1). A previous history of skin or throat infections or other viral infections may precede post-streptococcal glomerulonephritis or interstitial nephritis (see Table 1). Fever and altered mental status may be reported with the thrombotic angiopathies such as thrombotic thrombocytopenic purpura (TTP)/hemolytic uremic syndrome (HUS). HUS may be associated with a preceding gastrointestinal illness; a preceding history of bloody diarrhea a week prior is present in more than 80% of cases. Other abdominal symptoms include abdominal pain, nausea, and vomiting. New data is arising about atypical HUS (not associated with diarrhea) caused by mutations/inhibitors in the alternative complement pathways. Both TTP and HUS may have neurologic symptoms such as blurred vision, dysphasia, and memory loss. However, neurologic symptoms are less common in HUS. Fever, hemoptysis, and dyspnea may be reported with the pulmonary-renal syndromes such as Goodpasture's syndrome and the ANCA vasculitides (see Table 1). Henoch–Schonlein purpura (HSP) may have arthralgias, abdominal symptoms, and a purpuric rash (see Chap. 13 on "Dermatology").

4.3 Exam

Hypertensive emergency may be associated with renovascular injury. Fever is common with AIN, vasculitis, and TTP/HUS. Hypertension may be present with all intrinsic kidney diseases with glomerulonephritis along with edema in the hands and feet. Arthralgias may also be present with AIN, cryoglobulinemia, and HSP. Perseveration, agraphia, encephalopathy, and hyperreflexia may be present in TTP/HUS. Adventitious lung sounds may be present with the pulmonary-renal syndromes. The purpuric rash of HSP is usually found on the buttocks and lower extremities (see Fig. 1 in Chap. 13). A purpuric rash and signs and symptoms of peripheral neuropathy can be found in cryoglobulinemia. Purpura can also be found in lupus and the ANCA vasculitides.

4.4 Diagnostics

An extensive evaluation of glomerulonephritis is usually done as an inpatient often along with a renal biopsy. An ANA, Anti-dsDNA, ANCA, anti-GBM antibody, C3, C4, HIV, and hepatitis B and C are part of this work-up. Microangiopathic diseases are characterized by hemolytic anemia (elevated LDH and low haptoglobin) and thrombocytopenia. Proteinuria, pyuria, and hematuria are present in glomerulonephritis and red cell casts are pathognomonic. Pyuria is associated with tubulointerstitial disease and white cell casts are pathognomonic for this entity.

Key Points
- Hypertension and edema in the presence of a urinalysis with significant hematuria and proteinuria may represent glomerulonephritis.
- White cell casts are pathognomonic for tubulointerstitial disease. Red cell casts are pathognomonic for nephritic syndromes.
- Various systemic symptoms accompanied by renal failure with a new anemia and thrombocytopenia may represent microangiopathic hemolytic anemia (MAHA).
- MAHA requires hospital admission.

5 Post-renal Acute Kidney Injury

5.1 General Considerations

Post-renal AKI is caused by partial or total obstruction of urine drainage. This obstruction results in increased hydrostatic pressure within the urinary system and decreased glomerular filtration (GFR). Post-renal obstruction may occur anywhere along the urinary tract from the renal pelvis to the tip of the urethra. A bilateral process must be present above the bladder to cause significant differences in the GFR in the absence of a unilateral kidney or chronic kidney disease. These processes include retroperitoneal fibrosis, bilateral renal calculi, blood clots, or sloughed renal papillae such as from acute tubular necrosis (ATN). However, the obstruction most commonly occurs at or below the bladder neck. Common etiologies include benign prostatic hypertrophy, prostate cancer, neurogenic bladder, anticholinergic drugs or obstructed Foley catheters. Other causes of lower urinary tract obstruction are strictures, blood clots, and renal calculi in the bladder neck.

5.2 History

A history of infections may be present. A history of conditions associated with neurogenic bladder or medications such as anticholinergic drugs, or alpha-adrenergic antagonists (tamsulosin) may be elicited. A previous history of lower urinary tract symptoms may be present especially in males associated with prostatic hypertrophy. In post-renal AKI, pain in the abdomen or flanks is often present with rapid swelling of the drainage system. Flank pain only associated with voiding is pathognomonic for vesicoureteral reflux. A noticeable decrease in urinary volume (oliguria or anuria) may be reported (possible in all forms of AKI, but may be more sudden in post-renal AKI).

5.3 Exam

Suprapubic tenderness with a palpable bladder may be present if obstruction occurs at the bladder neck or urethra.

5.4 Diagnostics

The urinalysis may show pyuria and hematuria (stone disease) or bacteriuria (infection or colonization); however, the results are often normal. Ultrasound has an approximately 90% sensitivity for urinary tract dilatation (hydronephrosis/hydroureter) in post-renal AKI. False negatives may occur in the following cases: obstruction in the last 48 h, volume depletion, retroperitoneal fibrosis, or infiltrative disease. When obstruction is suspected, a significant increase in creatinine (decrease in GFR) implies total obstruction and should be referred to the ED.

Key Points
- History of flank and or suprapubic pain associated with a decrease in urine production is concerning for obstructive nephropathy.

- When post-renal AKI is suspected, a significant decrease in the GFR implies total obstruction and should be referred to the ED.
- An abdominal ultrasound is 90% sensitive for hydronephrosis which, if bilateral, needs a Foley catheter or other procedure for decompression.
- The placement of a Foley catheter, often in the ED, is required in cases of severe oliguria/anuria.

6 Renal Vein Thrombosis

Renal vein thrombosis is a deep vein thrombosis (DVT) in the renal vein that is frequently bilateral and results in acute kidney injury (AKI).

6.1 General Considerations

Renal vein thrombosis is a rare condition that can be either apparent or clinically silent. Two thirds of cases are bilateral and can result in AKI. Etiologies are typical for Virchow's triad: endothelial damage, venous stasis, or hypercoagulability. Virtually any hypercoagulable disorder can be associated with renal vein thrombosis, especially antiphospholipid syndrome and nephrotic syndrome. Those with severe nephrotic syndrome (massive proteinuria and hypoalbuminemia) are especially vulnerable. Other predisposing conditions are oral contraceptives, disseminated malignancy, factor V Leiden, and deficiencies in antithrombin and protein C and S.

6.2 History

Symptomatic renal vein thrombosis can be associated with flank pain.

6.3 Exam

Tenderness in the flank region may be present.

6.4 Diagnostics

The urinalysis may show hematuria and proteinuria. Doppler ultrasonography should be ordered in patients with renal failure at risk for thrombosis.

Key Point
- Patients with a history of a hypercoagulable state and renal failure should be evaluated with a Doppler ultrasound for renal vein thrombosis.

7 Electrolytes

7.1 Hyponatremia

Hyponatremia is generally a derangement of water balance relative to a stable salt homeostasis. Pseudohyponatremia may occur when there are extreme levels of glucose, lipids, or proteins in the serum. Severe elevations of proteins or lipids in the serum are characterized by a normal serum osmolality while hyperglycemia causes a hypertonic pseudohyponatremia (hyperosmolar hyperglycemia). A sodium of less than 130 is generally required to cause symptoms. These symptoms include headache, anorexia, nausea, disorientation, confusion, agitation, ataxia, and areflexia. When a sodium level is around 120 or less, more severe symptoms such as vomiting, seizures, coma, and ultimately cardiac arrest due to brain stem edema and herniation can occur. The exact laboratory value is of concern but also the rate of change plays a role in patient symptoms and ultimate disposition. Symptomatic patients with a sodium level less than 130 should be considered for referral for immediate labs, especially if they have no prior history of hyponatremia. In stable patients, hyponatremia may be evaluated with a repeat value and evaluations of urine and serum osmolality, urine sodium, and evaluations of adrenal, renal, cardiac, hepatic, and thyroid function. Hyponatremia is referred to as hypervolemic when associated with fluid overload. Hypovolemic hyponatremia is characterized by dehydration. Hypervolemic hyponatremia is often due to cardiac or hepatic dysfunction and results in edema and low urine sodium. Hypovolemic hyponatremia is usually due to fluid losses from vomiting, diarrhea, or diuretics and results in orthostasis or frank hypotension.

Normovolemic hyponatremia can be caused by a variety of factors such as ACE inhibitors and diuretics, adrenal and thyroid deficiency, hypokalemia, psychogenic polydipsia, and SIADH (syndrome of inappropriate antidiuretic hormone secretion). Renal dysfunction may be involved in hyponatremia regardless of fluid status (see Table 2).

Table 2 Etiology of hyponatremia delineated by volume status

Hypervolemic hyponatremia	Normovolemic hyponatremia	Hypovolemic hyponatremia
Congestive heart failure Cirrhosis	Medications (ACE inhibitors) Adrenal insufficiency Thyroid disease Hypokalemia Polydipsia SIADH	Vomiting Diarrhea Laxatives Diuretics

(Not an exhaustive list)
SIADH syndrome of inappropriate antidiuretic hormone

Key Points
- Symptoms of hyponatremia are not attributable to sodium unless the value is less than 130 mEq/L (usually significantly lower).
- Symptoms or signs should prompt immediate retesting either in the ED or outpatient lab depending on severity.
- A lab value of 125 mEq/L or less should be sent to the ED.

8 Hypernatremia

Hypernatremia is defined by a sodium greater than 145 and serum osmolality of greater than 305 and is relatively rare in outpatients. Like hyponatremia, hypernatremia may be hypervolemic causing edema, euvolemic (diabetes insipidus and hypodipsia), and hypovolemic causing orthostasis. Like hyponatremia, hypernatremia may cause nausea, vomiting, weakness, and lethargy. Polyuria is a common symptom of diabetes insipidus (greater than 3 L of urine per 24 h). When encountering hypernatremia, a repeated value with serum osmolality is appropriate in the absence of symptoms. Generally, symptoms are not apparent unless the level is 155–160 mEq/L. If there are symptoms, then a repeat measurement and exam should be repeated. Values equal to or greater than 155–160 mEq/L carry risk for seizure and should be referred to the ED. Patients with deranged drinking behaviors, CNS pathology affecting the thirst mechanism, or both are cause for concern in hypernatremia.

Key Points
- Hypernatremia is rare and symptoms generally do not occur unless the level is 155 mEq/L or more.
- Levels at or above this should prompt immediate evaluation. Levels greater than 150 mEq/L should be repeated and symptoms should be inquired about.
- Levels greater than 160 mEq/L should be sent to the ED.

9 Hypokalemia

Hypokalemia can be mild (3.0–3.5 mEq/L) or severe (less than 3.0 mEq/L). Mild hypokalemia is generally asymptomatic; however, a more significant decrease in potassium can lead to generalized symptoms of malaise and nausea with or without vomiting. Neurologic symptoms can present as paresthesias, muscle weakness and cramps, and eventually paralysis. Cardiac sequelae are the most serious and can lead to malignant arrhythmias and fatalities. EKG findings are flattened or depressed T-waves or prominent U-waves. The causes of hypokalemia are many, and gastrointestinal issues such as vomiting can make it difficult to distinguish between etiology and symptoms. Oral intake is a factor as hypokalemia is seen in eating disorders, starvation, and alcoholism. In alcoholism, hypomagnesemia can be found concurrently and worsens hypokalemia. Significant sweating can also result in hypokalemia. Intrinsic renal defects such as renal tubular acidosis (RTA) type I, often associated with Sjogren's (see intrinsic renal disease above), leads to hypokalemia. Cancer patients with hematologic malignancies can also develop hypokalemia due to RTA, and chemotherapy drugs can also cause hypokalemia. Medications such as diuretics are common causes. It should be noted that patients with recurrent hypokalemia, accompanied by alkalosis and elevated blood pressure (HTN) should undergo secondary HTN evaluation.

Key Points
- Hypokalemia can cause potentially fatal cardiac arrhythmias and patients with pre-existing heart disease are more susceptible.
- Severe hypokalemia is defined as less than 3.0 mEq/L.
- Healthy patients should be considered for ED referral at levels less than 2.5 mEq/L. Cardiac patients have a higher threshold.

10 Hyperkalemia

As an academic statement, hyperkalemia usually does not cause severe complications until the level is 7.0 mEq/L or above. However, in the outpatient setting, the results from the lab are delayed by 24 hours or more and the true level of the potassium is not known at the time of contacting the patient. Considering the potentially fatal consequences of a critically elevated potassium level, a potassium level above 6.5 should prompt immediate laboratory analysis in the ED and levels greater than 6.0 require immediate outpatient evaluation. The rapidity of increase is the concern and a rapid increase in the level of potassium causes more dramatic effects on cardiac muscle. In contrast, patients with chronic kidney disease can tolerate higher levels of potassium as their levels rise more gradually. The early EKG findings of hyperkalemia are peaked T-waves (only one lead is necessary) (see Fig. 3). Later, widening of the QRS complex is seen and malignant ventricular arrhythmias may result. In the outpatient setting, medications such as angiotensin converting enzyme (ACE) inhibitors or mineralocorticoid receptor antagonists especially when in combination are common culprits. Repeat labs may need to be performed to rule out pseudohyperkalemia. In vitro hemolysis results in a measured hyperkalemia and is accompanied by a raised AST in liver function tests (LFTs). Significant leukocytosis or thrombocytosis on the CBC can cause release of potassium by the same mechanism.

Key Points
- A potassium level of 6.5 mEq/L should be referred to the ED for monitoring and treatment.
- Patients with chronic renal failure and higher baseline levels of potassium can tolerate potassium levels and outpatient retesting may be appropriate.

11 Hypocalcemia

11.1 General Considerations

The physiological effect of hypocalcemia depends greatly on the rate of decrease of the calcium level. The most serious manifestations of hypocalcemia are neuromuscular and cardiac. Hypocalcemia causes irritability of all three forms of muscle, skeletal, cardiac, and smooth. Some symptoms such as weakness and fatigue are vague. Skeletal muscle cramps, tetany, and paresthesias can occur. Seizures can result from extremely low levels of calcium. Ventricular arrhythmias can result from the prolonged QT level seen on the surface EKG (see Fig. 3). Bradycardia, hypotension, and congestive heart failure are other cardiac findings. Smooth muscle effects are laryngeal spasm, bronchospasm, and respiratory failure. Other physical findings include generalized hyperreflexia, Chvostek sign (spasm with tapping of the jaw), and Trousseau sign (spasm of arm muscle with compression of the blood pressure cuff). Hypocalcemia can occur due to vitamin D deficiency, progressive renal failure, hypoparathyroidism, alcoholism, and hypomagnesemia. The serum calcium measurement may need to be corrected with the serum albumin. (For more information on hypocalcemia see Chap. 10 on "Endocrinology").

Key Points
- Severe hypocalcemia causes effects on neural and muscle tissue.
- Hypocalcemia can prolong the QT interval on the EKG.
- Levels less than 6.5 should be considered for referral to the ED.

12 Hypercalcemia

12.1 General Considerations

Mild hypercalcemia (less than 12 mg/dL) is usually asymptomatic. The symptoms of hypercalcemia are myriad and can affect almost any organ system. The most serious manifestations are cardiovascular with severe hypercalcemia causing arrhythmias including complete heart block. Calcium level should be corrected for albumin levels; and with milder elevations, an ionized calcium may be ordered. A calcium level greater than 14.0 mg/dL should generally be referred to the ED. The most common cause of this level of hypercalcemia is cancer for which an elevated calcium carries a poor prognosis. Other causes of hypercalcemia are medications such as thiazides, vitamin D toxicity, and granulomatous diseases. Granulomatous diseases cause an increase in the vitamin D3 level which is the mechanism for hypercalcemia. The rate of the increase of calcium in the serum is important in the evaluation and hyperparathyroidism is a common cause of a gradual, chronic rise in calcium levels. Chronically elevated levels of calcium can lead to progressive renal failure. (For more information on hypercalcemia see Chap. 10 on "Endocrinology").

Key Points
- A calcium level of 14.0 mg/mL should be referred to the ED.
- Most of the time, these levels are associated with a malignancy and carry a poor prognosis.

13 Hypomagnesemia

13.1 General Considerations

Hypomagnesemia can have various neuromuscular, cardiovascular, and gastrointestinal effects. Seizures and confusion can occur at extremely low levels. Cardiac manifestations include heart failure, dysrhythmias, and hypotension. Serious consequences usually do not occur until the serum concentration is less than 1.0 mg/dL. Oral intake is a common consideration and hypomagnesemia is often seen in those with malnutrition, eating disorders, and alcoholism. Vomiting and diarrhea can contribute. Proton pump inhibitors and loop diuretics are two medications commonly associated with hypomagnesemia. Hypomagnesemia exacerbates and propagates hypokalemia, and the potassium cannot be corrected until the magnesium is corrected. Similar is true with hypocalcemia.

Key Points
- Hypomagnesemia can cause seizures and arrhythmias.
- Serious complications do not occur usually until the level is less than 1.0 mg/dL.

14 Hypermagnesemia

14.1 General Considerations

Hypermagnesemia is a rare condition usually caused by increased intake of magnesium in the presence of chronic renal insufficiency or iatrogenic factors. Intake is usually accidental, often occurring with magnesium-containing laxatives or antacids. Symptoms of mild hypermagnesemia are nausea, vomiting, weakness, and flushing, which occur when the level is above 3 mg/dL. Diminishing of reflexes, hypotension and EKG changes can occur with levels between 4 and 5 mg/dL. The EKG changes consist of QRS widening, lengthening of the QT and PR intervals, and potentially dangerous conduction abnormalities and referral to ED for monitoring is appropriate at this level of magnesium. Coma, respiratory depression, and complete heart block occur at levels greater than 9 mg/dL, and cardiac arrest can occur at levels greater than 10 mg/dL.

Key Points
- Hypermagnesemia usually occurs accidentally due to ingestion of laxatives or antacids.
- Emergent referral for EKG monitoring occurs with levels greater than 4 mg/dL.

15 Hypophosphatemia

Hypophosphatemia symptoms are global and include lethargy, confusion, or disorientation. As with other ions, phosphate depletion causes neuromuscular effects and some symptoms mimic stroke such as dysarthria, dysphagia, oculomotor palsies, sensory deficits, and ataxia. Tremors and hyporeflexia are physical findings. Severe complications such as coma and seizures do not occur unless the level is less than approximately 1.0 mg/dL. Mild hypophosphatemia causes the common complaints of muscle weakness and bone pain. Hypophosphatemia generally occurs in hospitalized patients often with malignancy. Ambulatory patients often are malnourished with or without alcoholism or have intrinsic renal tubular defects such as seen in Sjogren's. Hypophosphatemia can occur as part of a refeeding syndrome in severely malnourished patients. Other causes are due to elevated PTH (hyperparathyroidism), PTH-related protein, or severe vitamin D deficiency.

Key Points
- Hypophosphatemia often occurs in malnourished or alcoholic patients or as a result of a refeeding syndrome.
- Neurologic effects including confusion, stroke mimics, and seizures, and usually do not occur until the level is 1.0 mg/dL or less.

Further Reading

Cydulka RK, Fitch MT, Joing SA, Wang VJ, Cline DM, Ma OJ, editors. Tintinalli's emergency medicine manual. 8th ed. New York: McGraw Hill; 2018.

Jameson JL, Fauci AS, Kasper DL, Hauser SL, Longo DL, Loscalzo J, editors. Harrison's principles of internal medicine. 20th ed. New York: McGraw Hill; 2018.

Levey AS, Bosch JP, Lewis JB. A more accurate method to estimate glomerular filtration rate from serum creatinine: a new prediction equation. Ann Intern Med. 1999;130(6):462–70.

Stevens L, Coresh J, et al. Assessing kidney function—measured and estimated glomerular filtration rate. N Engl J Med. 2006;354:2473–83.

Surawicz B, Knilans TK. Chou's electrocardiography in clinical practice. Philadelphia: W.B. Saunders; 2001.

Urology

Gregory M. Booth

1 Introduction

Emergencies of the urogenital system are examined in this chapter starting from the kidneys to emergencies of the male genitalia. Many of these are associated with extreme pain and will bypass the outpatient clinic; however, sometimes they will appear urgently or via a phone message to the clinician. Nephrolithiasis is extremely common and will occasionally be encountered in the primary care setting. As with all body systems, infections in locations that are anatomically confined and poorly accessible to immunologic defenses are prone to emergent complications such as Fournier's gangrene and prostatitis. When dealing with emergencies pertaining to male genitals such as testicular torsion, priapism and penile fracture, prompt effective management is extremely important as sexual and reproductive functions are at stake. Late complications of procedures and surgeries are covered briefly at the end of the chapter.

2 Nephrolithiasis

Nephrolithiasis is the formation of stones, or calculi, in the urinary tract.

G. M. Booth (✉)
Baltimore, MD, USA
e-mail: boothg444@yahoo.com

© The Author(s), under exclusive license to Springer Nature Switzerland AG 2022
G. M. Booth, S. Frattali (eds.), *Managing Emergencies in the Outpatient Setting*, https://doi.org/10.1007/978-3-031-15270-2_6

2.1 General Considerations

Nephrolithiasis (or urolithiasis) is extremely common with a lifetime risk of 12% for men and 7% for women. Most are caused by calcium oxalate stones.

Approximately 70% of stones occur in patients between the ages of 20 and 50. The number one risk factor for urolithiasis is previous stone formation. Thus, stone formation is uncommon in the elderly who have no prior history of urolithiasis. Other risk factors are dehydration, inflammatory bowel disease, bariatric surgery, hyperparathyroidism, diabetes, renal tubular acidosis, and gout. Calculi less than 5 mm have a 79–90% chance of passing spontaneously and may be treated medically with analgesics, antiemetics, and alpha-blockers such as tamsulosin. Stones greater than 5–6 mm have less than 50% chance of passing spontaneously within 7 days. Thus, a dedicated spiral CT to evaluate for stone size and other pathology should be ordered. Emergency conditions associated with urolithiasis are infection, obstruction resulting in severe hydronephrosis, and renal injury with an elevated creatinine. Pregnant patients should see a urologist promptly.

2.2 History

A history of renal failure, solitary kidney, or transplanted kidney should be inquired about, and, if present, lead to a more conservative course of action. Fever and chills may be present and indicate presence of infection which should be referred to the ED. Typically, patients with kidney stones will report sudden onset, severe, colicky flank or lateral abdominal pain radiating to the pelvis, inguinal area or groin. Nausea is extremely common.

2.3 Exam

Fever may be present. Costovertebral angle tenderness may be present and would suggest renal instead of solely ureteric involvement.

2.4 Diagnostics

Urinalysis is positive 85–90% of the time but may not be useful to determine the presence of infection versus simple stone disease. The presence of hematuria will wane over time. Renal failure in the setting of stone disease is concerning for bilateral urolithiasis and prompt imaging is necessary. Non-contrast spiral CT is the test of choice with approximately 95% sensitivity and specificity. The CT estimates the size and location of the stone which guides management decisions from a urologic perspective. In pregnancy, ultrasound is preferred to rule out obstruction but has lower sensitivity for detecting small stones.

Key Points
- The decision to refer to the ED is clinical taking into account ability to tolerate oral intake and pain control.
- The presence of fever with a clinical picture of kidney stone is concerning and should be considered for ED referral.
- Renal failure in the setting of urolithiasis requires prompt imaging and consideration of ED referral is appropriate.
- Nephrolithiasis in patients with a history of renal failure, solitary kidney, or kidney transplant needs a monitored setting.

3 Urinary Retention

Urinary retention is caused by failure of the bladder to empty resulting in pain and increased pressure throughout the urinary system.

3.1 General Considerations

Urinary retention is far more common in men occurring in approximately 5% of men throughout their lifetime due to prostatic hypertrophy. In both men and women, the etiology may be urinary tract infection, constipation, urethral stone or stricture, blood clots, or autonomic dysfunction. Also common to both males and females, medications are often implicated; examples are anticholinergics, anti-psychotics, and anti-Parkinson's drugs. In females, obstruction may occur due to organ prolapse, bladder procedures, or pelvic tumors. Urinary retention may rarely occur in a primary herpes simplex virus (HSV) infection and cause severe abrupt onset of symptoms associated with an active genital infection. Patients who experience an episode of obstruction will experience another within 6 months 20% of the time.

3.2 Causes of Urinary Retention

Males
- Prostatic hypertrophy

Females
- Organ prolapse
- Bladder procedures
- Pelvic tumors

Both males and females
- Constipation
- Urinary tract infection
- Urethral stone
- Urethral stricture
- Neurological conditions
- Recent surgery

Medications
- Anticholinergics
- Anti-psychotics
- Anti-Parkinson's drugs

3.3 History

The key symptom is an inability to urinate. Enquiries should be made concerning previous pelvic surgeries and urinary procedures. Patients with urinary retention are clearly uncomfortable, with symptoms usually occurring over hours as suprapubic pain and inability to urinate develop. Acute on chronic retention is often preceded by lower urinary tract symptoms such as urgency, frequency, and incomplete voiding. Fevers may be reported with an infection. The patient may also report constipation as the preceding symptom. Genital symptoms may be reported in genital herpes which is a rare cause of urinary retention in the young.

3.4 Exam

The bladder is often palpable in the suprapubic region. A prostate exam should be performed in men with obstruction. A rectal exam should be performed in patients with constipation to evaluate for impaction. A pelvic exam may be performed in women to assess for a mass as a cause for obstruction. Genital herpes can cause ulcerative genital lesions and an infectious proctitis that causes severe pain and fever. Inguinal lymphadenopathy often occurs with HSV.

3.5 Diagnostics

The urinalysis may be positive if urinary tract infection or urolithiasis are the causes. The patient will often not be able to give a urine sample.

Urology

Key Point
Patients with urinary retention are uncomfortable and have an inability to urinate in any appreciable amount. These patients need urgent decompression of the bladder in the ED.

4 Prostatitis

Prostatitis is a bacterial infection of the prostate gland.

4.1 General Considerations

Approximately, 80,000 cases of acute bacterial prostatitis occur annually. Prostate biopsy is the most common risk factor for bacterial prostatitis. Indwelling Foley catheters are the second most common risk factor for prostatitis. Other risk factors are obstruction of the lower urinary tract by anatomic or neurophysiological conditions. Ascending infection from epididymitis or urethritis, rectal intercourse, and phimosis are other common risk factors. The offending microorganism is usually *E. coli* with other Gram-negative urinary bacteria and *Staphylococcus* the remainder. Often, prostatitis can be managed effectively as an outpatient with sepsis, advanced age, immunocompromised status, including diabetes, as indication for consideration for ED referral.

4.2 History

Fevers may be reported. Pain in various locations such as the lumbar area, genitals, perineum, and suprapubic regions are commonly reported. Urinary complaints such urgency, frequency, and dysuria and pain with ejaculation are common. Decreased voiding or inability to void may be reported in cases of urinary obstruction and retention.

4.3 Exam

Fever may be present. The hallmark of infection is an exquisitely tender prostate on rectal examination. Vigorous manipulation of the prostate should be avoided as this increases hematogenous spread. Suprapubic or perineal tenderness is often elicited.

4.4 Diagnostics

The urinalysis and culture are usually positive, but a negative result does not exclude the diagnosis.

Key Points
- Prostatitis in patients with comorbidities can cause a quick onset of septic shock and observation is often required to ensure effectiveness of antibiotics.
- Negative urine studies do not rule out suspected acute bacterial prostatitis.

5 Fournier's Gangrene

Fournier's gangrene is a fulminant, necrotizing infection of the genital and/or perineal area.

5.1 General Considerations

Fournier's gangrene is an uncommon infection. The infection is polymicrobial consisting of Gram-negative (*E. coli, Klebsiella*), Gram-positive (Staphylococcal and Streptococcal spp.), and anaerobic (*clostridia*) microorganisms. Like necrotizing fasciitis (see Chap. 2 on "Infectious Emergencies"), early management is critical and includes surgical debridement. The infection arises from three sources: (1) skin, (2) genitalia, or (3) the colorectal route. Common sources from the skin are trauma, genital piercing, hydrocele aspiration, and vasectomy. Genital causes are genital infections, Foley catheter, urethral stricture, and incontinence. Colorectal causes are perirectal abscess, rectal biopsy, appendicitis, or diverticulitis. Patient risk factors are obesity, alcohol abuse, liver disease, decreased mobility, poor hygiene, and immunosuppression including diabetes and steroid use.

5.2 History

The history is similar to that of other severe infections. Fevers may be present. Any severe pain in the genitals, perineal, or low abdominal wall pain that represents a possible infection should be approached with a high index of suspicion for Fournier's gangrene.

5.3 Exam

The vitals should be appreciated. Elements of the systemic inflammatory response syndrome (SIRS) (see Chap. 2 on "Infectious Diseases", Table 1) are typically found to be elevated in Fournier's gangrene. Commonly seen in the elderly, incontinent, and immobile patient, a meticulous inspection of the perineal area should be made to avoid missing signs of this infection. Any blackening area of skin including the scrotum or perineum, or severe, tender, erythema in the pelvis and perineal area should raise concern for Fournier's gangrene.

5.4 Diagnostics

A CT scan can provide supporting information but the diagnosis is largely a clinical one.

Key Points
- Fournier's gangrene is an uncommon infection of the genital, perineal, and lower abdominal wall.
- The infection is necrotizing and any blackening of skin or severe painful erythema should raise concern for this condition.

6 Testicular Torsion

Testicular torsion is a twisting of the testicle about its axis that leads to irreversible testicular necrosis.

6.1 General Considerations

Most cases of testicular torsion occur in infants and adolescents; however, torsion can occur in any age group including very rarely in men over 40. Torsion is an emergency as it leads to veno-occlusion and arterial ischemia causing irreversible loss of reproductive germinal tissue.

6.2 History

A family history of torsion in the father or a brother may be reported. The typical history is a sudden onset of scrotal pain occurring in four different situations: (1) on awakening from sleep, (2) after strenuous exercise, (3) after trauma (even minor) to the genitals, or (4) after sexual activity. That being said, no preceding event may be related in cases of torsion, and torsion should be considered in any presentations of testicular pain. The patient may experience nausea and vomiting. The pain is felt in the lower abdominal quadrant, inguinal canal, or the testis itself, and is not positional. A gradual onset of pain would be very unusual and other diagnoses should be considered with such a history. Occasionally, patients report a suspicious history of previous intermittent symptoms and this is compatible with an impending permanent torsion. These patients should be sent to the ED. Sometimes, the patient will present a significant amount of time after the torsion event and be relatively asymptomatic resulting from infarction of the testicle as there is only a 6–8-hour window to salvage the testicle. At this point, the testicle should be emergently removed and the other fixed.

6.3 Exam

The patient should be examined both standing and supine. The patient suffering from torsion is in significant pain that is worse with movement and walks with a wide-based slow gait. In the upright position, the patient's testicle will be high riding and may be edematous and erythematous on inspection. Palpation may be accomplished with the patient supine and will reveal a tender testicle which is mildly enlarged, firm, and irregular. The cord structure will be difficult if not impossible to be palpated. The unilateral absence of the cremasteric reflex is a sensitive but not specific finding. An attempt can be made to manually accomplish testicular detorsion with a medial to lateral motion on the testicle similar to opening a book. If successful, emergency care is still required. Prehn's sign (relief of the pain on scrotal elevation) is not present with torsion as it is with epididymitis.

6.4 Diagnostics

In acute, highly suspicious cases, the Doppler ultrasound should not be ordered as this will delay a successful surgical outcome. If the Doppler is ordered, it will show no or decreased blood flow to the testicle; however, false negatives do occur and the diagnosis cannot be successfully ruled out with this modality. If a urinalysis is ordered, pyuria may be present and does not rule out testicular torsion.

Key Points
- A sudden onset of significant pain, to the point where gait is affected, is a typical history for testicular torsion.
- A high riding abnormal testicle with abnormal cord structures will help confirm the diagnosis.

- These patients require immediate tissue-saving surgery within a 6-hour time period. A Doppler ultrasound is unnecessary in cases with a convincing clinical picture.

7 Other Scrotal Pathology

7.1 General Considerations

Infections of the scrotum such as orchitis, scrotal abscess, and infected hydrocele can become problematic to the point of needing emergent care. Scrotal hematoma either from trauma or spontaneous often from bleeding diathesis or anticoagulation can on occasion need drainage emergently, and, likewise, hematomas can become infected. Orchitis or epididymitis in the younger patient is often sexually transmitted; however, in older patients the infection is usually from ascending Gram-negative bacteria. Bladder stasis from outlet obstruction is a common risk factor for such infections. Scrotal abscess and infected hydrocele almost always require drainage which is not usually done in the primary care office. The cause of a spontaneous scrotal hematoma should be investigated and coagulation profile should be drawn in patients taking coumadin. Whether the patient requires oral versus intravenous antibiotics or requires urgent versus emergent drainage depends on the severity of the condition and requires judgment. Quick availability of outpatient urology support often determines the ultimate disposition of the patient.

7.2 History

Risk factors for tuberculosis (see Chap. 2 on Infectious Emergencies Disease) should be kept in mind with scrotal infection not responding to antibiotics. A history of urinary retention or benign prostatic hypertrophy may accompany orchitis in the older patient. A sexual history should be taken in both younger and older patients. History of fevers may be reported and should be considered for escalation of care. Scrotal pain can be severe and also should be considered in the calculus for escalation of care.

7.3 Exam

Febrile patients should be referred for immediate care. In orchitis, the hemi-scrotum is usually erythematous and edematous and the infection may spread to the contralateral side. The scrotum and the perineum should be inspected for necrotic skin indicative of Fournier's gangrene (see above). In orchitis, the prostate should be evaluated for enlargement or abscess. The bladder should be palpated for distention. Trauma should be considered in hydrocele and scrotal hematoma.

7.4 Diagnostics

A scrotal ultrasound can evaluate whether a hydrocele is infected or not.

Key Points
- Systemic symptoms should prompt emergent management of scrotal infection.
- With scrotal infection, close inspection of the scrotum and perineum should be performed looking for necrotic skin indicative of Fournier's gangrene.

8 Priapism

Priapism is an unwanted erection lasting greater than 4 hours in the absence of sexual stimulation.

8.1 General Considerations

There are three types of priapism: (1) low flow (ischemic) (85%, of cases), (2) recurrent ischemic priapism (stuttering priapism), and (3) high flow priapism. Ischemic priapism is a true urologic emergency as greater than 4 hours of erection can cause permanent damage to the muscle and permanent erectile dysfunction (ED). The causes of priapism are numerous and include trauma to the area, spinal issues, and cancer in the penis or in the pelvis. Medications (phosphodiesterase-5 inhibitors, antidepressants, anti-psychotics, and anticoagulants) and toxins (alcohol, cocaine, and marijuana) can also cause priapism. Hematologic etiologies also are on the list especially sickle cell anemia. If the clinician receives a phone call from a patient with a prolonged erection, the patient can be instructed to run or perform some other adrenaline-producing exercise of the lower extremities as a temporizing measure. Patients with prescribed intracavernosal medications or devices can develop priapism. Those with devices may develop infections that require IV antibiotics and prompt urologic consultation.

8.2 History

The history is straightforward with a painful erection that lasts greater than 4 hours. Previous episodes and previous erectile function should be recorded. Meticulous documentation is required in the cases of prolonged erections to avoid litigation in poor outcomes.

8.3 Exam

The exam is also straightforward with an erect penis that spares the glans (rigid corpora cavernosa with a flaccid corpus spongiosum).

8.4 Diagnostics

A complete blood count and pelvic imaging are indicated for a patient with no active erection but a history of prolonged erections.

Key Point
- A patient with a prolonged (greater than 4 hours) painful erection should be referred to the ED for treatment and observation.

9 Miscellaneous

9.1 Penile Fracture

Penile fracture is a rupture in the tunica albuginea of the penis.

This uncommon injury is due to injury of the erect penis, most often during sexual activity. During erection the wall of the penis shrinks to 0.25 mm from 2 mm during the resting state reflecting its tensile strength. When a strong bending force is applied to the erect penis, rupture of the wall can occur usually at the ventrolateral aspect. Most men report sudden pain and an audible snap, pop, or crack and immediate detumescence though some erectile function may remain. Baseline erectile function should be documented as erectile dysfunction is a frequent complication. Urethral damage and hematuria are also common complications. The treatment for penile fracture is surgery within 24–36 h and the time of the incident and appointment in the clinic should be documented.

10 Surgical Complications

Ureteral injuries can occur due to any surgery in the pelvic region but commonly occur with gynecologic and bowel surgeries. Risk factors for ureteral injury during gynecologic procedures are prior pelvic surgeries, endometriosis, pelvic radiation, obesity, and fibroids.

10.1 History

The presentation is usually nonspecific with nausea, vomiting, fever, malaise with abdominal pain and distention.

10.2 Exam

Fever may be present. Urine is sterile so septic complications are rare but abdominal discomfort and distention may be present as chemical peritonitis can occur resulting in bowel dysfunction.

10.3 Diagnostics

Assessment of renal function is not sensitive enough to be useful for this condition and a CT urogram is the test of choice if this diagnosis is suspected.

Key Points
- High suspicion of ureteral damage must be held for patients with abdominal symptoms after recent gynecologic or bowel surgery.
- A CT urogram is the test of choice to confirm this diagnosis.

11 Cauda Equina Syndrome

Cauda equina syndrome is an emergency characterized by dysfunction of the sacral nerves resulting in low back pain, lower extremity numbness and weakness, and sudden onset of bladder, bowel and sexual dysfunction. The causes can be malignant or "benign." Benign causes include intervertebral disc rupture, spinal stenosis, spinal infection or hematoma, spinal trauma or fracture, and arteriovenous malformation. Malignant causes include primary spinal tumors or metastasis. Malignant causes will be covered in Chap. 11 on oncologic emergencies.

12 Complication of Lithotripsy

Lithotripsy is a common procedure and can often cause abdominal and flank pain, ureteral obstruction from fragments, gross hematuria, and skin ecchymosis. However, lithotripsy can cause emergent complications such as rupture or perforation of internal organs, vascular injury, pancreatitis, and severe infections. Perinephric and renal hematomas may also occur often associated with a new anemia and no hematuria on urinalysis. Infections include urosepsis, psoas abscess, and pyelonephritis. In stable patients, imaging and basic blood work may be pursued.

13 Complications of Ureteral Stents

A range of infections can occur after implantation of ureteral stents. These may or may not require a monitored setting and the urologist should be consulted in these cases. Sometimes the infections can be managed with oral antibiotics in the outpatient setting and stent removal is not necessary. Late complications can be seen with ureteral stents and new onset abdominal pain, flank pain, fever, symptoms of cystitis, or gross hematuria may indicate complications. These include stent migration, obstruction, or infection. A urinalysis should be obtained and imaging should be ordered to assess stent location. A new anemia in the absence of hematuria on urinalysis may indicate a hematoma. The urologist should be promptly notified in these situations. A vascular fistula can occur with an eroding stent and cause gross hematuria, hypotension, and syncope. These patients should be hospitalized immediately.

Further Reading

Cydulka RK, et al., editors. Tintinalli's emergency medicine manual. 8th ed. New York: McGraw Hill; 2018.
Goyal DG, Mattu A, editors. Urgent care emergencies: avoiding the pitfalls and improving the outcomes. New York: Wiley; 2012.
Snodgrass WT. Testicular torsion. In: Pediatric urology evidence for optimal management. Essay. Cham: Springer; 2013.
Thurtle D, et al., editors. Urologic emergencies. Lewisville: TFM; 2017.

Obstetrics and Gynecology

Gregory M. Booth

1 Introduction

Ectopic pregnancy and pelvic inflammatory disease are relatively common causes for abdominal pain in women of childbearing age. Most of the issues affecting pregnant patients discussed in this chapter are the domain of the patient's obstetrician. However, pregnant patients can be seen by their primary care clinicians for non-obstetric reasons or receive calls as a matter of urgency. Thus, primary care clinicians should be aware of obstetric emergencies.

2 Ectopic Pregnancy

Ectopic pregnancy is implantation of the products of conception outside of the uterus.

2.1 General Considerations

Ectopic pregnancy comprises 2% of all pregnancies, but the true incidence of ectopic pregnancy is hard to estimate due to underreporting of cases handled as an outpatient. Over 90% of ectopic pregnancies are fallopian; this is the most common site causing severe complications, as over 95% of deaths in ectopic pregnancy are due to a tubal rupture. Risk factors for ectopic pregnancy are outlined in Table 1 with

G. M. Booth (✉)
Baltimore, MD, USA
e-mail: boothg444@yahoo.com

Table 1 Risk factors for ectopic pregnancy

Risk factors for ectopic pregnancy
Intrauterine device (IUD)
Prior infection (PID)
Prior ectopic pregnancy
Prior abdominal surgery
Tubal sterilization
Infertility
Increasing age
Endometriosis
Prior spontaneous abortion
Ovulation induction
Smoking
Pelvic tuberculosis
Pelvic schistosomiasis

PID pelvic inflammatory disease

intrauterine device (IUD), prior ectopic pregnancy, prior infection, and prior surgery including tubal ligation highlighting the list. Around one-third of pregnancies following sterilization are ectopic. The use of emergency contraception has not been found to be a risk factor for ectopic pregnancy.

2.2 History

Abdominal pain (90%), vaginal bleeding (50–80%), and amenorrhea (70%) are the classic triad of symptoms for ectopic pregnancy. The pain is a vague lower abdominal pain that may become sharp and crampy as tubal distension occurs. As stated, amenorrhea is classically reported; however, a different menstrual history may be described, such as a lighter or abnormally timed period. If there is a ruptured tubal pregnancy, there may be shoulder or upper abdominal pain due to stimulation of the phrenic nerve by a hemoperitoneum.

2.3 Exam

Vital signs may be, but not always, abnormal with significant bleeding, and orthostatic blood pressures should be performed. Orthostatic blood pressures are defined by a 20 mmHg drop in systolic or a 10 mmHg drop in diastolic blood pressure 30 seconds after arising from a supine to a standing position. The pelvic pain is typically unilateral but can be bilateral or contralateral to the side of the ectopic pregnancy. Rebound and guarding are unusual. The utility and safety of a pelvic exam has come into question in recent medical discourse; however, the exam may reveal cervical motion tenderness, adnexal tenderness with or without a mass, and vaginal bleeding which can be light or heavy.

2.4 Diagnostics

A urine pregnancy test has a high sensitivity for pregnancy and is virtually 100% accurate for a symptomatic ectopic pregnancy. However, a false negative test can sometimes be found with extremely dilute urine. In this case, a serum pregnancy test should be ordered.

Key Points
- Any non-pregnant patient with abdominal pain and a positive pregnancy test should be referred to the ED for evaluation of ectopic pregnancy.
- In stable patients with minimal symptoms and an unclear diagnosis, a serum pregnancy test may be ordered.

3 Ovarian Torsion

Ovarian torsion is a twisting of the ovary on its pedicle resulting in vascular obstruction.

3.1 General Considerations

Torsion is infrequent but not uncommon, with approximately 3% of surgical emergencies in women carrying this diagnosis. Any suspicions of this diagnosis should be closely evaluated, as a classical presentation only occurs 50% of the time. The risk factors include young age, history of ovarian cysts, current pregnancy, or use of reproductive technologies. Though typically a condition of premenopausal women, a female of any age can be affected. The anatomy is a twisting of the infundibulopelvic ligament around its axis. The predominance of torsed ovaries is on the right side perhaps because of stabilization of the infundibulopelvic ligament by the sigmoid colon. Over half of the affected ovaries either had a dermoid cyst (38%) or a hemangioma (24%), and another 20% were from a serous adenoma or a corpus luteum. The diagnosis is difficult to make clinically, and even imaging has been found to be often non-diagnostic. As stated below, the pain is typically of sudden onset, but case series have shown that patients often present after 7–8 days of symptoms.

3.2 History

The most common complaint is pelvic pain. Classically the onset of pain is sudden; however, more than half the time this does not occur, often causing delays in diagnosis. The next most common symptom is nausea with or without vomiting occurring about 2/3 of the time. The abdominal pain is usually unilateral, but up to a quarter of cases are bilateral. One half of patients have radiation of pain to the back, flank, or groin, often brought on by exertion. Some patients have very mild symptoms.

3.3 Exam

Abdominal exam will usually reveal unilateral tenderness and peritoneal signs may be present. The pelvic exam reveals unilateral adnexal tenderness and a palpable mass representing the inciting cause such as a cyst.

3.4 Diagnostics

An ultrasound will show a mass in all patients. Doppler evaluation can be helpful and shows a twisted vascular pedicle in the majority of cases. However, Doppler flow may be normal due to twisting and untwisting of the ligament. Further evaluation with CT or MRI is useful in some cases.

Key Points
- In a patient with sudden abrupt unilateral pelvic pain with associated nausea, ovarian torsion should be ruled out.
- An ultrasound will show a mass in all cases.
- Subtle presentations are possible and interruption of Doppler flow is not always present at time of ultrasound study.

4 Pelvic Inflammatory Disease

Pelvic inflammatory disease (PID) is a spectrum of infections of the upper female reproductive tract, most commonly caused by *N. gonorrhoeae* or *C. trachomatis*.

4.1 General Considerations

Approximately 200,000 PID cases occur each year with many patients treated in the outpatient setting. Though common, PID often does not follow the typical pattern of symptoms and a high suspicion must be held for this diagnosis. PID comprises endometritis, salpingitis, tubo-ovarian abscess, and pelvic peritonitis. Risk factors include young age (teenagers are at most risk), multiple sexual partners, a new sexual partner within the last 30 days, history of sexually transmitted disease, and intrauterine device (IUD) insertion within the previous 3 weeks. Mild symptoms and signs may be managed with oral antibiotics; however, concern for tubo-ovarian abscess usually mandates same day imaging. If outpatient treatment is pursued, follow-up within 72 h is recommended. A common outpatient treatment is ceftriaxone 250 mg IM × 1 plus doxycycline 100 mg bid × 14 days plus metronidazole 500 mg bid × 14 days. In a small minority of patients, a syndrome of perihepatitis called Fitz-Hugh and Curtis syndrome is found which can mimic cholecystitis. PID patients may need to be hospitalized, especially pregnant women, HIV positive patients, adolescents, and those who are unable to arrange follow-up within 48–72 h.

4.2 History

Many women with PID have non-specific or very subtle symptoms. The most common presenting symptom (reported 90% of the time) is lower abdominal pain. The pain can be reported as generalized. Other symptoms are vaginal discharge (75%), vaginal bleeding preceding or coincident with the pain (40%), and urinary symptoms (20%). Systemic symptoms such as fevers and nausea with or without vomiting make the diagnosis of tubo-ovarian abscess clearer. Rarely, pleuritic right upper quadrant pain can be reported with liver inflammation (perihepatitis).

4.3 Exam

Fever may be present but is not necessary for the diagnosis. The hallmark findings are uterine or adnexal tenderness or cervical motion tenderness on pelvic exam. Mucopurulent vaginal discharge is often found, and samples are sent to the lab for analysis. In more severe cases, signs of peritonitis are found with rebound tenderness. Right upper quadrant pain, often pleuritic, can be reported with perihepatitis.

4.4 Diagnostics

A pregnancy test is mandatory in premenopausal female patients with abdominal pain. If feasible, the same day imaging may be accomplished with pelvic and transvaginal ultrasound to rule out abscess. Elevated white blood cell count is present 60% of the time and increased sedimentation rate is found 75% of the time. Liver enzymes will be normal in perihepatitis as the liver parenchyma is not inflamed.

Key Points
- Fever and pelvic pain in a sexually active female should raise suspicion for tubo-ovarian abscess which requires same day imaging.
- Urinary symptoms may be present and also, rarely, liver involvement.
- A pregnancy test should always be obtained in a premenopausal woman with abdominal pain to evaluate for ectopic pregnancy.

5 Vaginal Bleeding

Vaginal bleeding will be divided into two categories: bleeding in the pregnant versus non-pregnant patient.

5.1 Vaginal Bleeding in the Non-pregnant Patient

5.1.1 General Considerations

Menorrhagia and metrorrhagia are now subsumed under the term abnormal uterine bleeding (AUB). AUB can occur anytime throughout the menstrual cycle. Postmenopausal bleeding is rarely an emergency (some advanced cases of vaginal cancer are an exception) and will not be covered. The etiology for abnormal uterine bleeding is now divided into the PALM–COEIN classification system based on the acronym PALM for structural disorders and COEIN for non-structural disorders (Table 2).

Table 2 The PALM–COEIN classification for abnormal uterine bleeding (AUB)

Structural	Functional
Polyp	Coagulopathy
Adenomyosis	Ovulatory dysfunction
Leiomyoma	Endometrial
Malignancy and hyperplasia	Iatrogenic
	Not classified

5.1.2 History

Historical elements include timing of bleeding, any endocrine conditions, and medications such as antiplatelet or anticoagulants. Other questions regarding propensity to bleed are appropriate in the evaluation, as up to 20% of patients with AUB have a coagulopathy. Inquiring about past treatment for anemia, heavy bleeding after other procedures such as dental work or childbirth or surgeries is also appropriate. Epistaxis, bleeding from cuts for longer than 5 min, or frequent bruising greater than a quarter in size are common. The passing of clots greater than a quarter during menses is also a risk factor. Any family history of the above is a consideration as von Willebrand disease is common in AUB. A thorough sexual history should also be obtained as sexual trauma especially with sex toys can precipitate vaginal bleeding in patients. The most important clinical finding is the patient reporting the use of one or more pads or tampons per hour as they are at risk for decompensation.

5.1.3 Exam

The volume status of the patient should be established with orthostatic blood pressure measurements. A drop of 20 mmHg in systolic or 10 mmHg in diastolic blood pressure 30 seconds after standing from a lying position qualifies as orthostasis though smaller deviations may be significant. A pelvic exam should be performed and active red bleeding arising from the cervical os implies potential vascular compromise. If the blood is dark red, not arising from the os, and does not pool, the bleeding is likely non-emergent.

5.1.4 Diagnostics

A pregnancy test should always be performed and it should be recalled that the urine pregnancy test is not 100% sensitive. A complete blood count can be drawn in less emergent conditions to assess for chronic blood loss requiring transfusion.

Key Points
- Patients who are using one or more pads per hour during an episode of vaginal bleeding are at risk for decompensation.
- A pregnancy test should be performed.
- A complete blood count can be obtained for chronic cases.

5.2 Vaginal Bleeding in the Pregnant Patient

5.2.1 General Considerations

The first step in diagnosing a pregnant patient with vaginal bleeding is to determine whether the patient is carrying an intrauterine pregnancy. Once an ectopic pregnancy is ruled out, then the patient can be advised that bleeding in the first trimester is not uncommon. Up to 15% of women who deliver term pregnancies report some amount of bleeding up to 14 weeks into the pregnancy. However, it is crucial to rule out any other underlying problems before assuming the best. According to data from the World Health Organization, 1/3 of pregnancies will spontaneously abort, approximately 75% of those being in the first 8 weeks of pregnancy. As such, first trimester bleeding in the stable patient should be followed closely with the obstetrician. In contrast, bleeding during the second and third trimesters of pregnancy implies a significant and urgent complication, often involving abnormalities of the placenta or placental abruption. Uterine rupture can also occur, especially in patients with previous cesarean sections and in women with short interdelivery interval. Trauma, even minor, can be associated with abruption of the placenta. A placental abruption is characterized by painful vaginal bleeding. In all cases, vaginal bleeding in all pregnant patients is managed in close coordination with their obstetrician as it may portend significant bleeding complications or threatened abortion.

5.2.2 Exam

In pregnancies at approximately 20 weeks or less, a pelvic exam showing an incompetent cervix denotes inevitable abortion. A digital exam is contraindicated in patients with placenta previa.

5.3 Vaginal Bleeding After Elective Abortion

5.3.1 General Considerations

A patient who has received an elective abortion may experience emergent vaginal bleeding. Elective surgical abortion is a common procedure with approximately one million performed every year. Hemorrhage complicates 1 out of every 20 abortions as a result of retained products, uterine atony or rupture, cervical laceration, or perforation. Medical abortions are accomplished by oral mifepristone followed by misoprostol buccally 24–48 h later. Medical abortions, now more common than in previous decades, comprised approximately 1/3 of abortions performed in 2014. Very rarely, 1 in 30,000 spontaneous pregnancies, an intrauterine pregnancy is accompanied by an ectopic pregnancy. This is termed heterotopic pregnancy, which is frequently accompanied by continued symptoms following the abortion. Heterotopic pregnancy is even more common in an in vitro fertilization, occurring in 1/100 pregnancies.

5.3.2 History

In both threatened and elective abortions, a thorough obstetrical history should be obtained with number of vaginal and caesarian deliveries, plus elective and spontaneous abortions reported. A medical abortion will be accompanied by several hours of heavy bleeding and cramping which, although possibly severe, should resolve within 24 h. Symptoms beyond this timeframe should prompt concern. The physician should inquire about history of fever or chills to assess for septic abortion. The physician should also ask the use of anticoagulants including aspirin. Abdominal pain may be associated with uterine rupture; however, rupture is not always associated with severe pain.

Key Points
- Vaginal bleeding during the second and third trimesters is always pathologic and requires prompt evaluation by the obstetrician.
- Bleeding 24 h after a planned abortion also requires prompt evaluation.

6 Pre-eclampsia

Pre-eclampsia is a disorder of unknown etiology that causes widespread organ dysfunction in pregnant patients.

6.1 General Considerations

Pre-eclampsia and eclampsia are generally the domain of the patient's obstetrician; however, the primary care physician should be aware of this condition. Hypertensive disorders of pregnancy are common, found in up to 10% of patients. The risk factors include previous pre-eclampsia, multifetal pregnancy, diabetes, obesity, extremes of maternal age, nulliparity, and triploidy in the fetus. Included in the definition of pre-eclampsia is the presence or absence of severe factors; however, the patient with any degree of pre-eclampsia may rapidly decompensate. The diagnosis is defined by elevated blood pressures in the presence of proteinuria after the 20th week of pregnancy. It should be noted that the proteinuria associated with pre-eclampsia is extremely variable, so one urinalysis cannot definitely rule out the presence of pre-eclampsia. Hypertension is the most reliable finding in pre-eclampsia. Defined as a blood pressure equal to or greater than 140/90 found on two readings 4 hours apart, potentially pre-eclamptic patients should be referred to the hospital for further evaluation. Relative elevations in blood pressures should be noted in patients where previous data is available. For example, a blood pressure of 130/80 in a patient with a baseline blood pressure of 100/60 is concerning. The HELLP syndrome is characterized by the presence of *h*emolysis, *e*levated *l*iver enzymes, and *l*ow *p*latelets and is a variant of pre-eclampsia that may be present without proteinuria.

6.2 History

The patient may report rapid weight gain (approximately 2 pounds in a week) and edema. Headache, blurry vision, shortness of breath, and epigastric pain are often reported, usually late in the course.

6.3 Exam

The blood pressure should be elevated above 140/90 or significantly above the patient's baseline. Epigastric or right upper quadrant tenderness may be elicited in those with HELLP syndrome. Edema in the face and/or hands is common. Hyperreflexia at the knees can be appreciated.

6.4 Diagnostics

Proteinuria, defined as 1+ on a urine dipstick, is diagnostic.

Key Points
- In a pregnant patient beyond the 20th week without a previous diagnosis of hypertension, a sustained blood pressure equal to or greater than 140/90 should be referred for immediate evaluation.
- Both weight gain and proteinuria define the disorder but are not always present together and should not impede continued evaluation in concerning cases.

7 Hyperemesis Gravidarum

Hyperemesis gravidarum (HG) is nausea and vomiting in pregnancy that results in dehydration and vascular instability.

7.1 General Considerations

Nausea and vomiting is present 60–80% of the time in the first 12 weeks of pregnancy. However, the clinician should have awareness for more serious etiologies of vomiting despite its common nature. HG is not usually associated with abdominal pain and its presence should elicit consideration for intra-abdominal pathology. The differential is extensive and includes gastrointestinal causes (peptic ulcer disease, gastroenteritis, etc.), pancreatitis, hepatobiliary disease, appendicitis, and pyelonephritis. Unstable vital signs and ketonuria are the keys to diagnosing HG in an outpatient setting. HG is treated with intravenous (IV) fluids.

7.2 History

Fever and abdominal pain indicate a different diagnosis. Nausea and vomiting are definitive.

7.3 Exam

Hypotension or orthostasis indicate need for IV fluids. Orthostasis is defined by a 20 mmHg drop in systolic blood pressure or 10 mmHg drop in diastolic blood pressure upon raising the patient from a lying to a standing position, 30 seconds should elapse after the maneuver before blood pressure is taken.

7.4 Diagnostics

The presence of ketonuria confirms HG; and, when significant, provides evidence for the need of IV fluids. Electrolyte abnormalities are common as well.

Key Point
- Hyperemesis gravidarum is defined by unstable vital signs or ketonuria and these patients often require IV fluids in the ED if the vomiting cannot be controlled.

8 Sexual Assault

8.1 General Considerations

Unfortunately, sexual assault or rape is a common crime. According to The Bureau of Justice Statistics, there were 431,840 rapes and sexual assaults in the USA in 2015. However, accurate statistics are difficult to obtain; most rape victims who know their assailants do not report the crime to the police. It also should be noted that approximately 5–10% of rape victims are men. A clinician's job, when encountering a patient who was sexually assaulted, is to provide support and refer them to the appropriate authorities and mental health specialists. If the assault was recent enough (1 week) that physical evidence may be present, the patient should be referred to the ED or other emergent setting, such as a rape crisis center for management.

Further Reading

Benrubi GI, editor. Handbook of obstetric and gynecologic emergencies. 5th ed. Baltimore: Wolters Kluwer; 2020.

Cydulka RK, Fitch MT, Joing SA, Wang VJ, Cline DM, Ma OJ, editors. Tintinalli's emergency medicine manual. 8th ed. New York: McGraw Hill; 2018.

Goyal DG, Mattu A, editors. Urgent care emergencies: avoiding the pitfalls and improving the outcomes. New York: Wiley; 2012.

Otolaryngology (Ear Nose and Throat)

Ioan A. Lina and Mark F. Williams

1 Introduction

The conditions in this chapter focus on the structures of the ear, nose, and throat involved in potential emergent pathophysiology. Epistaxis is covered first as the most commonly encountered otolaryngology-related issue in primary care. Infections of the throat and neck follow (peritonsillar and retropharyngeal abscesses, Lemierre's syndrome, and epiglottitis). The emergent ear infections of mastoiditis and malignant otitis externa are covered subsequently. A discussion of peripheral versus central vertigo addresses the discernment between benign and emergent causes of vertigo in the ambulatory patient. Sudden sensorineural hearing loss and the rare emergent complications of acute rhinosinusitis are covered last.

2 Epistaxis

Epistaxis is a common complaint in both the outpatient and emergency settings. While nose bleeds are often self-limited, severe epistaxis can be seen in 0.2% of patients and can result in life threatening hemorrhage and may require urgent intervention. Understanding the etiology, anatomical location, and associated comorbidities in patients with epistaxis is essential for effectively triaging and providing excellent care.

I. A. Lina · M. F. Williams (✉)
Department of Otolaryngology - Head and Neck Surgery, The Johns Hopkins University School of Medicine, Baltimore, MD, USA
e-mail: Ilina1@jhmi.edu; markfwilliamsmd@yahoo.com

2.1 General Considerations

In advance of laboratory data, clinical history and physical exam will dictate urgency of evaluation and further treatment. The patient should be promptly evaluated for active signs of bleeding and potential for airway compromise. Patients who are incapable of protecting their airway due to loss of consciousness or severe neurological trauma (GCS <8) should proceed with intubation prior to nasal intervention. Moreover, systemic signs of hemodynamic instability including pallor, dry mucous membranes, tachycardia, orthostatic hypotension, or loss of consciousness, often indicate the need for urgent evaluation and intervention. Therefore, accurately quantifying volume of bleeding is essential. At greater than 100 mL of blood loss, visual estimation has been demonstrated to be grossly inaccurate amongst both medical and non-medical personnel. However, as a general reference, the U.S. cup contains 236 mL of fluid. The availability of low continuous wall suction can therefore be beneficial for patient comfort and quantification of active bleeding. While there is no global definition for severe epistaxis, bleeding of greater than 500 mL is often concerning due to changes in hemodynamic stability. Moreover, the UK epistaxis audit reviewed 1826 cases of epistaxis and defined severe bleeding as lasting greater than 30 min over a 24-h period.

2.2 History

A thorough history with regard to medications, social practices, and medical conditions should be obtained. Common etiologies can include digital or other trauma (such as nasogastric tube insertions), mucosal irritation and dryness, or use of steroid nasal sprays. However, less common etiologies should also be considered such as septal perforation, substance use, sinonasal cancer, arteriovenous malformations, and autoimmune-related disorders (such as granulomatosis with polyangiitis or immune thrombocytopenic purpura). Severe epistaxis also can be associated with medical conditions such as renal failure, hepatic failure (especially with alcohol), hypertension, and diabetes. Congestive heart failure is a common risk factor due to increased pressures in the vascular supply to the nose. A family history of bleeding disorders can also prompt the need for further testing for inherited diseases such as Von Willebrand's disease or other hemophilia. It is also important to elicit a thorough history including prior epistaxis, use of antiplatelet, or anticoagulation medications. Easy bruising, skin rashes such as petechiae or purpura, or bleeding after wisdom teeth extractions are also suspicious features for bleeding diathesis. Recurrent epistaxis may also be suspicious for malignancy in patients with other risk factors such as tobacco use, radiation or wood dust exposure, or prior history of nasopharyngeal cancer. Intranasal drug abuse can also present with recurrent epistaxis and potential septal perforation secondary to avascular necrosis of the septal cartilage. These medical conditions are important in evaluating patients with epistaxis as they give prognostic information as to whether the bleeding will be controlled in the clinic.

2.3 Exam

If the patient is actively bleeding, having the patient gently blow into a tissue can allow better evaluation of the nose. Anterior rhinoscopy with use of a nasal speculum (if available) should be performed on all patients with active epistaxis in conjunction with a use of a light source such as a headlight or otoscope as it may provide direct visualization of the source of bleeding. Often an area of bleeding or clot in the anterior nares in Kiesselbach's plexus can be appreciated in anterior epistaxis. However, the nasal floor, inferior and middle nasal turbinates and lateral nasal wall should also be examined carefully. Bleeding from both nares, hematemesis, or the presence of dark, melanotic stools may represent posterior epistaxis which may require additional packing or specialized intervention.

2.4 Diagnostics

In general, the treatment of epistaxis in the majority of patients is performed prior to obtaining laboratory information. In patients taking anticoagulation, a PT/INR may be necessary for determining if the patient is in a supratherapeutic window which may require correction. A CBC can also be helpful in estimating blood loss, specifically when trended over a period of time. While there is generally no role for imaging unless for preoperative planning purposes. Other testing will depend on the history obtained from the patient (autoimmune work up, malignancy workup, etc.).

2.5 Treatment

Treatment of epistaxis can be divided into two primary types based on anatomic location: anterior or posterior. Anterior epistaxis is by far the most common and can often be controlled in an outpatient setting in an otherwise healthy patient. Treatment of anterior epistaxis includes the use of 5–6 sprays of oxymetazoline (if available) in each nares coupled with firm constant pressure of the alar cartilages against the septum for 20 min without alleviation. Providers may therefore find it effective to concurrently perform a review of the patient's medical history during this time.[1] In general, care should be taken to refrain from inserting foreign materials into the nares as these may cause further mucosal trauma, may become foreign bodies, or may shunt bleeding into the posterior oropharynx. Cessation of bleeding usually indicates that a clot has formed, and further intranasal intervention should be avoided. To promote mucosal healing following cessation of bleeding, the patient

---

[1] Caution should be taken in patients with severe pulmonary hypertension which may be exacerbated by oxymetazoline.

should use an intranasal saline spray or spray-gel to prevent drying of the mucosa or clot.

Due to its location, posterior epistaxis arising from the posterior septum, nasopharynx, and posterior turbinates are unlikely to be effectively treated with vasoconstrictive nasal sprays and anterior nasal pressure. In these cases, referral to the otolaryngology office or ED for insertion of packing material in the posterior nose and nasopharynx is typically performed using non-absorbable packing material. Specifically, the use of double balloon catheters (anterior and posterior) was shown effective in controlling up to 70% of patients with posterior epistaxis. Otolaryngology should usually be consulted in most cases of severe posterior epistaxis to evaluate if there is need for additional intervention.

Recurrent epistaxis or epistaxis which is refractory to pressure and vasoconstricting agents may require additional interventions such as chemical cauterization, placement of absorbable or non-absorbable intranasal packing, or operative intervention. If utilized, packing should be inserted as atraumatically as possible. While there is no standard for the duration of packing, it is typically recommended that packing should remain no longer than 5 days. The use of tetracaine spray or lidocaine infused lubricants may make packing more tolerable in patients.

Key Points
- Bleeding from bilateral nares and large amounts of blood (>500 cc) originating from the posterior oropharynx may be indicative of posterior epistaxis which often needs to be managed in the ED.
- Patients encountering epistaxis with multiple medical comorbidities which is intractable to pressure and intranasal oxymetazoline often cannot be managed in an outpatient clinical setting.
- Patients on coumadin may need to be referred to the ED for a stat PT/INR.

3 Peritonsillar Abscess

Peritonsillar abscess (PTA) is a polymicrobial bacterial infection in the parapharyngeal space of the oropharyngeal cavity. Although patients may be toxic appearing, if treated effectively, the majority of patients will often make a speedy recovery.

3.1 General Considerations

The overall incidence for patients developing a PTA is 30 cases/100,000 people per year. The incidence of PTA often increases from childhood to peak in adolescents and young adults with subsequent decline amongst older adults. While there is no statistical association between the incidence of PTA's with seasonal variations, anecdotally most providers feel that there is an increase in the fall and winter time associated with the increased incidence of group A strep pharyngitis infections.

3.2 History

A comprehensive history is critical for elucidating between acute pharyngitis, tonsillitis, malignancy, and peritonsillar abscess. Patients with a PTA will often present with a history of worsening unilateral sore throat, dysphagia, odynophagia, and upper respiratory infection symptoms which have developed over the course of several days. Classically, patients may have a muffled "hot potato" voice, though more subtle voice changes can be found. Fevers and chills are also often reported along with malaise. As the abscess progresses, patients may subsequently develop worsening trismus (secondary to inflammation of the pterygoid muscles) and ear pain (referred pain). In addition, it is also critical to establish if the patient has trialed oral antibiotics and for what duration. Peritonsillar abscesses are almost exclusively characterized by their unilateral behavior. While bilateral PTAs are described, the presence of bilateral tonsillar swelling and/or exudates are likely indicative of acute pharyngitis which can be managed more conservatively.

3.3 Exam

A full and detailed head and neck exam is essential for the appropriate diagnosis of PTA.

The most common exam finding is displacement of the uvula away from the affected side with obvious mass effect of the affected tonsil which is displaced medially and anteriorly. The exam may be limited by reduced mouth opening. Therefore, a headlight and multiple stacked tongue depressors may be beneficial to open the mouth sufficiently in order to obtain an accurate exam. Care should be taken to assess the floor of mouth and submandibular region to rule out other potential sources of infection. Lymphadenopathy of the submandibular and upper cervical lymph nodes of the ipsilateral neck may also be present. However, bilateral lymphadenopathy with exudative tonsillitis should raise the suspicion for mononucleosis.

3.4 Diagnostics

A CT scan is 100% sensitive for a peritonsillar abscess. If aspirated, culture data is critical for ensuring appropriate antibiotic selection if there is recurrence.

3.5 Treatment

The primary treatment of a peritonsillar abscess involves antibiotics and steroids +/− drainage as dictated by exam and imaging findings. Antibiotic selection should take into account if the patient has failed outpatient therapy and if there is high concern for a drug resistant organism. Augmentin is often an excellent choice in patients with prior history of failure on amoxicillin or clindamycin. In the emergency room setting, patients often report significant symptomatic improvement following Intravenous dexamethasone, particular in the cases of odynophagia with poor PO intake.

Drainage of a peritonsillar abscess is typically performed in the ED or ENT office. Patients who are refractory to initial medical management or with imaging suggestive of a >2 cm abscess typically are taken for surgery. Drainage often includes needle aspiration and/or a stab incision which provides a pathway for egress. Cultures of the aspirated fluid is critical for future antibiotic selection, particularly when there is concern for recurrence.

Key Points
- A peritonsillar abscess is characterized by a markedly painful antero-medially displaced tonsil with deviation of the uvula away from that tonsil.
- In cases of doubt, a CT scan can rule out the diagnosis.
- Peritonsillar abscesses often require drainage which can be safely performed in the ENT clinic or emergency room setting in most cases.

4 Retropharyngeal Abscess

A retropharyngeal abscess is a rare but critical deep neck infection which arises posterior to the deep cervical fascia in a potential space which extends from the skull base to the posterior mediastinum. The retropharyngeal space contains two lymph node chains which typically drain the nasopharynx (including adenoids), paranasal sinuses, middle ear, and Eustachian tube.

4.1 General Considerations

Retropharyngeal abscess occurs mainly in children less than 5 years of age but in rare cases it can occur in adults. Infections are often found to be polymicrobial. Additional concern for pharyngeal injury or trauma secondary to foreign bodies (fish bone) or iatrogenic procedures (such as endoscopy, nasogastric tube insertion, and intubation) may also result in the development of a retropharyngeal abscess.

Otolaryngology (Ear Nose and Throat)

4.2 History

In the majority of cases, patients typically present following a several day history of upper respiratory illness. Symptoms such as severe sore throat, odynophagia, dysphagia are often common along with fever and chills. As the abscess progresses, patients may go on to develop nuchal rigidity, neck tenderness, drooling, and ultimately respiratory distress. Changes in voice may also be reported. Patients with high suspicion for retropharyngeal abscess should be managed in the emergency room setting.

4.3 Exam

The patient may have a fever and be toxic appearing. They will also often be uncomfortable. Signs of acute distress such as stridor, tripoding, or increased respiratory rate should prompt urgent consultation with otolaryngology for possible intervention.

4.4 Diagnostic Testing

CT neck with contrast is useful for determining the extent of abscess formation and can guide the operative approach for intervention. In the absence of a CT, lateral soft tissue radiograph is a quick and easy study to evaluate for RPA in patients who are otherwise stable. A CBC and blood cultures may also be useful.

4.5 Treatment

Prompt initiation of IV antibiotics is essential for treating patients with retropharyngeal abscesses. Similar to other abscess, antibiotic selection is essential and a detailed history of prior antibiotic use elucidates concerns for antibiotic resistant organisms. In otherwise stable patients, failure for improvement over 24–48 h typically will prompt the need for possible surgical drainage with otolaryngology.

Key Point
- Patients with retropharyngeal abscess are typically young children who present with severe throat pain which can progress to airway compromise. Treatment is typically performed in an emergency medicine setting and requires prompt initiation of antibiotics.

5 Lemierre's Syndrome

First described in 1936, Lemierre's syndrome occurs typically in response to oropharyngeal infections and is characterized by thrombophlebitis of the internal jugular vein with possible metastatic septic emboli and bacteremia.

5.1 General Considerations

The condition is rare with an annual incidence of 3.6 cases per one million people with the majority of cases occurring in patients between the ages of 14 and 24, with a possible male predominance. Lemierre's syndrome is caused by members of the normal oropharyngeal flora and the most common pathogen is *Fusobacterium necrophorum*. Other infections besides pharyngeal infections can cause Lemierre's including dental infections, sinusitis, otitis media, and parotitis. The onset is usually 1–3 weeks after the original infection. While the exact mechanism has not been fully elucidated, it is hypothesized that infection of the oropharynx extends into the lateral pharyngeal space resulting in direct or hematogenous spread to the internal jugular vein.

5.2 History

Fever and neck pain may be reported. A history of concurrent or preceding infection of the head and neck is often reported and in most cases is related to pharyngeal infection. Historical elements of pulmonary complications such as cough, hemoptysis, shortness of breath, and pleuritic chest pain are common. The joints are also commonly affected causing arthralgias and arthritis. Visceral abdominal internal abscess may also occur in liver, spleen and kidney.

5.3 *Exam*

Tenderness over the neck is the most common finding. The angle of the jaw or the area of the sternocleidomastoid may also be affected. Erythema, swelling, and induration may be present over these areas. Of note, almost half of patients may not have neck findings on presentation. If there has been spread to other organs then abnormalities of exam of those organs may be present. Adventitious lung sounds may be present. Abdominal or flank tenderness may be present with abscesses of internal organs. Moreover, a careful neurological exam is necessary to evaluate for possible development of intracranial abscesses.

5.4 Diagnostics

A CT of the neck with contrast is the study of choice. A carotid ultrasound may also be ordered but is less sensitive. The chest is the most common site of septic emboli deposition and a CT with contrast is the test of choice.

5.5 Treatment

The use of antibiotics including beta-lactamase inhibitors is essential. While there is no consensus for the use of anticoagulation in patients with Lemierre's syndrome, the risks and benefits should be considered prior to its use. Surgical intervention is often limited.

Key Points
- Lemierre's syndrome is an uncommon infection of the internal jugular vein usually after an oropharyngeal infection.
- In up to half of cases, the neck has minimal or no symptoms.
- The lung is the most common site of embolization and symptoms commonly arise from this organ system.
- A multidisciplinary approach is essential to prevent and treat septic shock and embolic spread to other organ systems.

6 Epiglottitis

Epiglottitis is a rare bacterial infection of the tissues of the neck surrounding the glottis.

6.1 General Considerations

Epiglottitis also known as supraglottitis is now rare following routine vaccination of children against *H. influenzae* type B; however, cases can still occur in adults due to *Streptococcus* and *Staphylococcus* species and waning immunity or lack of vaccination. Epiglottitis can occur at any age and in the older age groups the presentation may be more subtle. Risk factors are immunodeficiency including HIV and diabetes, end-stage renal disease, and substance abuse.

6.2 History

Fevers may be reported. The cardinal symptom of both epiglottitis and retropharyngeal abscess is a severe sore throat. A change in voice quality may be reported.

6.3 Exam

The patient may have a fever and be toxic appearing. Often the patient will be anxious and appear uncomfortable. A telltale sign of epiglottitis is marked tenderness with manipulation of the hyoid bone and a normal appearing oropharynx. In the later stages, the patient may be in a tripod or sniffing position due to respiratory distress. Care should be taken with any manipulation of the airway including use of a tongue depressor due to concern for laryngeal spasm. The patient often cannot control secretions or stridor may be present.

6.4 Diagnostics

Radiographs will not typically be ordered as an outpatient; however, lateral neck radiographs of epiglottitis typically show the thumbprint sign of a swollen epiglottis.

Key Points
- Both retropharyngeal abscess and epiglottitis are associated with severe throat pain.
- A reported severe throat in the absence of oropharyngeal erythema and with marked tenderness with manipulation of the hyoid bone should raise concern for epiglottitis.
- If symptoms are accelerating, emergency services may need to be called.

7 Mastoiditis

Mastoiditis is a serious infection of the mastoid cavity (a portion of the temporal bone) which is typically a complication of progressive otitis media.

7.1 General Considerations

Acute otitis media is an infection of the middle ear space, which is bounded by the tympanic membrane (ear drum), cochlea and labyrinth medially, mastoid cavity superoposteriorly, and Eustachian tube anteroinferiorly. The middle ear space communicates with the mastoid air cells via the antrum which allows for the potential spread of serous fluid or infection. Although extremely rare, complications of acute otitis media can include meningitis, epidural abscess, petrous apicitis, the development of abscesses, or lateral sinus thrombosis.

7.2 History

Often there is a history of preceding URI symptoms or several days of current symptoms leading to the diagnosis of otitis media. Patients will often subsequently develop fevers. Symptoms of otitis media are present such as otalgia, hearing loss, tinnitus or vertigo. Patients may have also failed more conservative measures.

7.3 Exam

The patient may be febrile. The TM may be bulging and erythematous with purulence visualized behind the TM. Hearing is often reduced in the affected ear. Erythema and/or tenderness of the postauricular skin is the tell-tale sign of mastoiditis and must be examined in every patient. When severe, this can result in protrusion of the auricle due to edema. The cranial nerves should be assessed to address concern for intracranial extension. Abscess eroding through the sternocleidomastoid muscle, known as a Bezold abscess, may also be seen as a rare complication.

7.4 Diagnostics

A CT scan may be performed, but it is important to note that fluid in a mastoid cavity alone is not sufficient for the diagnosis of mastoiditis. Mastoiditis is a clinical diagnosis. If CT is performed, many people with allergic rhinosinusitis or who have had a recent URI, will have transient fluid in their mastoid cavities. Specific signs of mastoiditis, however, include erosion of the bony septae between air cells, erosion of the outer cortex of the mastoid cavity, extracortical spread of infection or abscess into the sternocleidomastoid muscle, or signs of dural thickening or inflammation. Blood markers for infection such as ESR and CRP are also usually elevated.

7.5 Treatment

The treatment of mastoiditis includes the prompt administration of IV antibiotics and typically surgical intervention with at least the placement of a pressure equalizing tube and/or mastoidectomy.

Key Points
- Mastoiditis is characterized by fever, a protruding auricle and mastoid tenderness.
- A CT can confirm the diagnosis if there is erosion of bony septae, however, fluid alone is not indicative of mastoiditis.

- Mastoiditis is an invasive infection that requires IV antibiotics and urgent otolaryngology consultation.

8 Malignant Otitis Externa

Malignant otitis externa is a severe bacterial infection of the external tissues of the ear canal often invading the mastoid or temporal bone (osteomyelitis).

8.1 General Considerations

Malignant otitis externa is usually due to progressive otitis externa ("swimmers ear") which spreads to the bony–cartilaginous junction of the external auditory canal. Malignant otitis externa is most common in patients with diabetes mellitus, the elderly, and patients who are immunocompromised. Organisms are varied and may include fungal organisms, especially when topical antibiotic drops have been previously used. However, the majority of cases are caused by *Pseudomonas aeruginosa*. The preceding infection of otitis externa is also known as swimmer's ear: however, there are other risk factors besides swimming, including use of ear plugs, dermatitis in the ear, use of cotton swabs, and use of chemicals near the ear such as hair dyes and sprays.

8.2 History

The typical presenting symptom is out of proportion pain in the ear canal and conchal bowl which is worsened with touching the ear itself. Patients will often state that they are unable to sleep or use a cell phone to that side. Other symptoms can include headache or earache with vertigo or hearing loss. It is important to assess the patient's past medical history including prior use of topical or enteral antibiotics, control of their diabetes, and recent use of other immunosuppressant medications such as steroids.

8.3 Exam

Pain with manipulation of the auricle is almost always present. The finding of black colonies (aspergillus) or white patches (candida) can lead to a diagnosis of fungal origin. The external auditory canal is typically erythematous and can be swollen. Patients will often have difficulty tolerating otoscopy examination. If visible, involvement of the bony–cartilaginous junction of the external auditory canal is pathognomonic for malignant otitis externa.

8.4 Diagnostics

A CT of the temporal bone is the most sensitive modality for evaluating the external auditory canal. Cultures can be useful in cases of persistent disease to rule out multidrug resistant pseudomonas.

8.5 Treatment

Topical anti-pseudomonal ear drops with steroid in the case of bacterial infection +/− oral antibiotics vs. topical antifungal ear drops with steroid. Possible placement of an ear wick to ensure antibiotic penetration in the setting of canal edema. Prompt serial otolaryngology examination for serial debridement.

Key Points
- Malignant otitis externa is a contiguous osteomyelitis caused by a severe otitis externa infection.
- Risk factors are age, uncontrolled diabetes, and immunosuppression.
- Long term IV antibiotics are required (at least 6 weeks) usually with serial arthroscopic debridement and topical antimicrobial drops.
- CT can confirm the diagnosis.

9 Vertigo

Vertigo, or the sensation of imbalance secondary to vestibular dysfunction, is one of the most frequently encountered otolaryngology related pathologies. Vestibular vertigo is thought to account for 25% of dizziness complaints and occurs in about 1.4% of the population each year.

9.1 General Considerations

In general, there are two types of vertigo: peripheral vs. central.

9.1.1 Peripheral Vertigo

Many common etiologies of peripheral vertigo include benign paroxysmal positional vertigo (BPPV), vestibular neuronitis or labyrinthitis, otitis media, trauma, Meniere's disease, superior semicircular canal dehiscence syndrome, or toxin induced. *Labyrinthitis* will typically present with both auditory and vestibular dysfunction and can be secondary to viral or bacterial infections and induce inflammation of the inner ear. It can also result in acute sensorineural hearing loss

(SNHL). *Vestibular neuronitis* on the other hand typically results in vestibular dysfunction alone and is thought to be secondary to a viral infection of the vestibular nerve and vestibular apparatus. In viral etiologies, patients may often present with a URI prodrome. As the most common cause of non-infectious peripheral vertigo, *BPPV* occurs secondary to displacement of otoliths within the vestibular canals which stimulate one, if not more, axis of movement in sudden bursts. Although *Meniere's disease* is less common, it typically is associated with aural fullness, fluctuating SNHL, tinnitus, and intermittent vertigo (drop attacks). In the setting of trauma, a full work up should be performed to evaluate for evidence of violation of the otic capsule or labyrinth as these can precede a perilymph fistula.

9.1.2 Central Vertigo

Central causes of vertigo can include neurological disorders (multiple sclerosis, Parkinsonism, seizure, stroke, vascular insufficiency, cerebellar lesions, metabolic disorders, intoxication, migraine, and iatrogenic). Acute persistent severe vertigo, particularly in the setting of additional neurologic deficits, should be considered a stroke until proven otherwise. Multiple sclerosis and other neurological disorders can also present with additional neurological findings in the absence of a cerebral vascular event. Symptoms which are progressive over several months and associated with headaches or intraocular papilledema may suggest the presence of a cerebellar pontine angle tumor.

9.2 History

Asking the patient to describe specific sensations is paramount to ensure appropriate diagnosis and treatment. Patients with vertiginous sensations will describe active movements such as "spinning" or "whirling." Disequilibrium on the other hand is often described as feeling "off-balance." Whereas people with presyncope will often use words such as feeling "lightheaded" or "faint."

The onset and duration of symptoms is also paramount. Vertiginous symptoms that are seconds to minutes are often associated with BPPV or vascular insufficiency whereas hours of vertigo symptoms are more often associated with Meniere's disease or migraine. Vertigo related to vestibular neuronitis or labyrinthitis can typically last days given its inflammatory etiology whereas constant vertigo which is not relieved with positioning or time is likely related to a central etiology. Other components include the presence of otitis media, aural fullness, tinnitus, and hearing loss which are also important particularly when preceded by a history of recent URI symptoms.

9.3 Exam

In the case of infectious etiologies, fever may be present. The findings of otitis media may be present. Nystagmus may be present with both labyrinthitis and vestibular neuronitis. A full neurological exam should be performed on any patient presenting with acute vertigo symptoms. A HINTS exam (head impulse, nystagmus, and test of skew) is also useful for differentiating between central and peripheral vertigo. A Dix–Hallpike exam (lying the patient down while supporting their head and having them fix their eyes) can be helpful to diagnose BPPV and should elicit gaze-evoked rotatory nystagmus towards the side of the stimulus lasting 10–60 s with vertigo.

9.4 Diagnostics

Neurological examination with a head CT with thin cuts through the temporal bone can be a useful first step. Additional imaging can include an MRI brain as well as MRA (magnetic resonance angiography) if there is high suspicion of stroke or vascular insufficiency. Outpatient testing using videonystagmography (VNG) and audiogram can also be helpful for monitoring persistent deficits.

9.5 Treatment

Treatment varies based on the etiology of vertigo. Diagnosis is critical for appropriate treatment of patients with vertigo.

Key Points
- Vertigo is complex yet can be divided into central and peripheral causes.
- Rapid neurologic examination and imaging to rule out neurovascular compromise is essential.
- While acute labyrinthitis secondary to otitis media may require use of antibiotics, steroids can otherwise be beneficial to abate inflammatory causes of vertigo.

10 Sudden Sensorineural Hearing Loss

Sudden sensorineural hearing loss should be considered a medical emergency and requires prompt examination to rule out stroke and traumatic etiologies of hearing loss.

10.1 General Considerations

Sudden sensorineural hearing loss (SSNHL) is characterized by acute sensorineural hearing loss occurring over at least three consecutive test frequencies and developing over a 72-h period. Approximately 5–20 per 100,000 people per year in the USA are afflicted and there is no sex predisposition. Any age can be affected by SSNHL, though incidence in middle age is most common. SSNHL is almost always unilateral and most cases are idiopathic. Recovery of hearing depends on the severity and etiology of the hearing loss, however, there is often a worse prognosis if associated with vertigo, deafness, or a delay in treatment initiation. When identified, infectious (viral, lyme disease, and syphilis), and otologic etiologies occur most frequently. Primary otologic etiologies, most often medications (loop diuretics, sildenafil) are also very common. However, SSNHL can be related to neoplastic (masses, hyperviscosity syndrome), Neurologic (stroke, multiple sclerosis) and metabolic syndromes (diabetes), and autoimmune diseases and vasculitis. The latter two are often most frequently encountered in the case of bilateral SSNHL, although rare. Unfortunately, in the majority of SSNHL a definitive cause is never identified.

10.2 History

Patients will typically present with sudden loss of hearing upon waking or that progressively worsens throughout the day. This is sometimes perceived as a fullness or blockage of the affected ear and therefore patients may defer evaluation. History of concurrent URI may suggest acute otitis media. More than 90% of patients with SSNHL will have ipsilateral tinnitus and a large percentage will have vertigo. A previous history of such symptoms or fluctuating symptoms may lead to a diagnosis of Meniere's disease the evaluation of which is not urgent. Pain is occasionally reported or paresthesias. Hearing loss associated with other symptoms such as headache or diplopia may indicate a neurovascular etiology and require urgent imaging. Recent head trauma, barotrauma, or noise exposure can also cause abrupt hearing loss and a history of these factors can obviate the need for extensive urgent evaluation. If there is a tympanic membrane rupture, associated with noise or barotrauma the patient should be instructed regarding strict water precautions and follow up with expedited ENT referral.

10.3 Exam

The external ear canal should be inspected in addition to the tympanic membrane. A painful ear should not be irrigated if cerumen impaction is present. If the primary care clinician cannot manually dis-impact the ear, a referral to ENT is appropriate. A full neurological exam should also be performed. The clinician must make every effort to discern conductive from sensorineural hearing loss. In this regard, a tuning fork (512 Hz) can be used in the performance of the Weber test. In the Weber test, the struck tuning fork is placed midline (such as the forehead) and the sound will lateralize away from the affected ear in sensorineural hearing loss. A Rinne test (testing between air or in front of the ear vs. bone conduction, placed on the mastoid bone) will often be equivocal in the case of SNHL.

10.4 Diagnostics

Testing should be tailored to the clinical scenario. Some testing commonly utilized is complete blood count and metabolic panel (multiple myeloma, diabetes), inflammatory markers (ESR and CRP) for autoimmune diseases and vasculitis. An ANA is typically part of the evaluation. Consideration for an MRI of the brain should be had in all cases.

10.5 Treatment

Early initiation of steroids with either 60 mg oral prednisone daily (in adults) and/or with intratympanic injections, for a minimum of 10–14 days increases the rate of spontaneous recovery in SSNHL. Patients will often demonstrate the greatest recovery in the first 2 weeks.

Key Points
- Sudden sensorineural hearing loss (SSNHL) is defined as sudden hearing loss occurring over 72 h or less.
- While most cases are idiopathic, evaluation should be tailored to the clinical scenario.
- Otolaryngology evaluation for intratympanic steroid injections should be a consideration, and for cases of possible SSNHL where cerumen is unable to be manually disimpacted by the primary care clinician.

11 Acute Rhinosinusitis

Diagnosis of *acute rhinosinusitis* (*ARS*) is based on the sudden onset of >2 nasal symptoms for a duration of up to 12 weeks. While rare, complications of sinusitis can be severe and life threatening.

11.1 General Considerations

The prevalence of rhinosinusitis in the general population varies from 6 to 15%. Complications of sinusitis can be grossly classified as either extracranial or intracranial. Extracranial complications are from infection of the sinuses which spread to the premaxillary subcutaneous tissue, forehead overlying the frontal sinus (Pott puffy tumor), and extending into the eye. The Chandler classification is useful for categorizing ophthalmologic complications and include: preseptal cellulitis, postseptal cellulitis, subperiosteal abscess, orbital abscess, and cavernous sinus thrombosis. Cavernous sinus thrombosis shares some symptoms with orbital cellulitis which most often arises from the posterior ethmoid or maxillary sinuses (see Chapter on "Ophthalmology"). These often require joint evaluation by both otolaryngology and ophthalmology to ensure source control and eye integrity. Intracranial complications include epidural and subdural abscesses, superior sagittal sinus thrombosis, and meningitis. Epidural abscess is the most common intracranial complication and most likely arises from ethmoid or frontal sinusitis. While usually benign, mucoceles can become mucopyoceles and cause osteomyelitis or intracranial abscesses. Patients with poorly controlled diabetes or other immunosuppressive states may be susceptible to additional complications of infection, including development of invasive fungal sinusitis.

11.2 History

The history is typical for a non-resolving acute rhinosinusitis. Significant fevers may be reported which are uncommon for rhinosinusitis. Pain is often referred to the eye and forehead with epidural abscess. Cavernous sinus thrombosis can cause visual impairments such as double vision. Fever and pain over the frontal sinus are consistent with Pott's puffy tumor requiring IV antibiotics.

11.3 Exam

Significant fever, eye pain, and sinusitis should raise concern for an emergent complication. Cranial neuropathies especially of cranial nerve six and proptosis should be referred to the ED. Necrotic or darkened nasal turbinates in diabetics or immunosuppressed patients should be referred for emergent care to rule out possible invasive fungal sinusitis.

Otolaryngology (Ear Nose and Throat)

11.4 Diagnostics

Thin cut (~1 mm) CT with contrast is an effective first diagnostic test for identifying complications of sinusitis. In the case of concern for intracranial complications, MRI can be more sensitive for identifying dural inflammation and perivascular invasion. Purulence emanating from the middle meatus warrants culture.

11.5 Treatment

Prompt initiation of IV antibiotics is imperative in the treatment of complicated ARS. Otolaryngology and/or ophthalmology consultation is often necessary to ensure appropriate source control. Invasive fungal sinusitis is often life threatening and involves serial debridement of the sinuses.

Key Points
- The presence of significant fever or an abnormal neurological exam in cases of sinusitis should raise concern for an emergent complication.
- Mold visualized as darkened or black spots on the turbinates in poorly controlled diabetic or immunosuppressed patients should be referred to the ED to rule out invasive fungal infection.

12 Miscellaneous

12.1 Foreign Bodies

12.1.1 General Considerations

Foreign bodies in the ear, nose, and throat are commonly encountered in the primary care setting.

12.1.2 Ear

Foreign bodies in the ear can often be removed by the primary care clinician using an otoscope and forceps or a suction catheter. Insects may be immobilized with the installation of lidocaine. Extreme care should be taken to avoid trauma of the canal wall skin and the tympanic membrane. Foreign bodies which are visualized to perforate the tympanic membrane warrants otolaryngology evaluation give the risk of injury of the ossicles and/or the inner ear. Clear fluid draining from the perforation may suggest a perilymphatic fistula. Following removal, ear drops containing an antibiotic and steroid should be prescribed for 5 days to ensure canal wall healing following trauma.

12.1.3 Nose

A frequent event in children, patients will often present after multiple attempts from the parents which inadvertently lodges the object more posteriorly. Most foreign bodies can be visualized on anterior rhinoscopy and can be removed with the assistance of Bayonette forceps or soft-catheter suction if available. Utilizing oxymetazoline (if available) is essential to provide decongestion and enlarge the nasal passage to facilitate removal. A Fogarty balloon can also be an effective tool for removal of foreign bodies if available. Care should be taken not to cause trauma to the nasal septum or head of the turbinates as this can result in bleeding making it more difficult for future attempts at removal. If unable to remove, the patient should be given nasal saline spray and a prophylactic antibiotic to protect against toxic shock syndrome with subsequent referral to an otolaryngologist.

12.1.4 Throat

Particularly in children, stridor, dyspnea, tachypnea, changes in voice, and tripoding are concerning for migration into the airway and require urgent bronchoscopy and evaluation for removal. In adults, patients will classically present with having a "fish bone" stuck in the throat. AP and lateral XR of the neck can be useful for identified foreign objects when radiopaque. In most cases, a foreign body is not identifiable in which case otolaryngology consultation is needed for flexible fiberoptic laryngoscopy. In children, the presence of a button battery (seen as two concentric rings on XR) should be treated urgently as battery acid leakage may erode through the esophagus into the neck.

Further Reading

Barkwell D, Arora R. Labyrinthitis. Treasure Island (FL): StatPearls Publishing; 2021.
Bontempo LJ, Shoenberger J, editors. Ear nose and throat emergencies. Amsterdam: Elsevier; 2019.
Cydulka RK, Fitch MT, Joing SA, Wang VJ, Cline DM, Ma OJ, editors. Tintinalli's emergency medicine manual. 8th ed. New York: McGraw Hill; 2018.
Dalrymple SJ, et al. Tinnitus: diagnosis and management. Am Fam Phys. 2021;103:663–71.
Goyal DG, Mattu A, editors. Urgent care emergencies: avoiding the pitfalls and improving the outcomes. New York: Wiley; 2012.

Pulmonology

Gregory M. Booth

1 Introduction

Pulmonary embolism (PE) and community acquired pneumonia (CAP) are covered in the cardiovascular and infectious disease chapters respectively. Asthma and COPD are extremely common conditions that often present in an emergent fashion to the primary care setting. Interstitial lung disease is a group of rare conditions that occasionally present with exacerbations. Massive hemoptysis will occasionally be reported and should be referred to the ED. Hemoptysis in lesser amounts may also be part of a syndrome (i.e., tuberculosis or PE) that requires an ED referral. Pleural effusion is common and requires urgent attention when causing symptoms or when a malignant effusion needs to be ruled out. Pneumothorax will occasionally present to the clinic and needs radiographic confirmation and aspiration in the ED.

2 Asthma and COPD

Asthma and chronic obstructive pulmonary disease (COPD) are two diseases of the airways that can lead to severe hypoxia and death.

2.1 General Considerations

Asthma and COPD are two extremely common lung diseases that are characterized by exacerbations with significant morbidity and mortality. Although asthma and COPD have very different etiologies, approximately 10–15% have an asthma/COPD overlap syndrome. Asthma is generally a disease of triggered airway constriction, in a patient with a predisposition to the disease based on various factors that are endogenous (genetic) and environmental. Triggers include allergens, exercise, cold air, infections among others. COPD is generally a more persistent, chronic condition with various degrees of airway inflammation and destruction from tobacco smoke. In young patients with COPD, an alpha-1 antitrypsin level is checked for any link to this treatable genetic disorder (alpha-1 antitrypsin deficiency). Diagnosis of COPD is aided by pulmonary function tests (PFTs) which reveal a persistent airflow limitation. Asthma is also diagnosed by PFTs which reveal airway limitation reversed by a beta-agonist. The variability in asthma pathology and symptoms sometimes requires a methacholine challenge which is often not done in clinical practice. The treatment of asthma and COPD is similar with inhaled beta-agonists, inhaled corticosteroids, and inhaled anticholinergic medications as the mainstay of chronic treatment. In end-stage COPD, oxygen therapy is used to improve quality of life and mortality from right sided heart failure due to hypoxic pulmonary vasoconstriction. Exacerbations are commonly treated with oral corticosteroids and a nebulized beta-agonist (albuterol) with or without an anticholinergic (ipratropium). At times, exacerbations are severe and the patient needs to be sent to the ED for continuous nebulizer treatments and intravenous (IV) steroids.

2.2 History

In asthma exacerbations, common triggers such as indoor and outdoor allergens should be evaluated. Passive exposure to fumes including cigarette smoke are also triggers for asthma. The presence of an infection is a common precipitant to both asthma and COPD. Shortness of breath and wheezing are the most common complaints in asthma and COPD. COPD exacerbation is defined by the presence of cough and sputum production or increased cough and increased sputum production. Fatigue is commonly reported with both conditions. Altered mental status due to narcosis is sometimes encountered.

2.3 Exam

As in other causes of lung dysfunction, pulse oximetry in severe exacerbations will often be low at less than 93%. Patients with COPD may have chronically low pulse oximetry readings. Sometimes the pulse oximetry will be normal and the patient's status will be revealed by the respiratory rate (RR). A RR of greater than 30 is considered a relative indication for intubation so careful attention to this vital sign should be recorded and plays a role in the calculus for patient disposition. Adventitious breath sounds are the hallmark of both asthma and COPD. Wheezing and rhonchi are found in all lung fields, often in the upper chest near the bronchi in asthma. In severe exacerbations of both asthma and COPD, bronchoconstriction can be so severe that marked decrease of breath sounds will be heard and this is an ominous sign. The presence of crackles argues against the diagnosis of asthma or COPD and suggests congestive heart failure, pneumonia, or interstitial lung disease.

2.4 Diagnostics

The chest radiograph in both asthma and COPD will be either normal or show hyperinflation without other abnormalities.

2.5 Treatment

In most offices, a nebulizer treatment will be available and can prevent the ED referral of a patient who does not have nebulizers at home.

Key Points
- Severe exacerbations of asthma and COPD sometimes require continuous inhaled nebulizers and IV steroids.
- Age, comorbidities, pulse oximetry, and respiratory rate are considered when referring the patient to a higher level of care.

3 Interstitial Lung Disease

Interstitial lung disease is a heterogeneous group of disorders that affect the lung parenchyma due to inflammation and fibrosis.

3.1 General Considerations

Interstitial lung disease (ILD) is a large heterogeneous group of chronic lung disorders that generally cause progressive symptoms. The progressive nature of these disorders does not lead to a referral to the ED typically, and the evaluation for these disorders occurs as an outpatient. However, exacerbations do occur and require hospitalization on occasion. A full treatment of ILD is beyond the scope of this book, but some comments will be made. Smoking and male sex are risk factors for the most common ILD, interstitial pulmonary fibrosis (IPF) which has a poor prognosis. Autoimmune diseases that are associated with ILD include myositis which can be associated with cancer. Medications such as nitrofurantoin and those associated with treatment of rheumatologic disorders (methotrexate, azathioprine, rituximab, and the TNF-alpha blockers) can cause ILD. Sarcoid is a very common disease that causes ILD. Cryptogenic organizing pneumonia (COP) mimics an infection and can be idiopathic or associated with connective tissue disease or cancer.

3.2 History

A history of connective tissue disorders should be elicited. The performance of a social history of smoking and environmental exposures is pertinent. The typical symptoms are a dry cough, dyspnea on exertion, and fatigue. Chest pain is uncommon but can be reported with sarcoid. Hemoptysis is uncommon. Raynaud's phenomenon may be reported in autoimmune disorders such as lupus.

3.3 Exam

Tachypnea, tachycardia, and a decrease in pulse oximetry may be present. Cyanosis on the lips and fingertips may be present. Clubbing may be present. Wheeze is uncommon and the typical finding is fine inspiratory crackles at the bilateral bases.

3.4 Diagnostics

A chest radiography may be abnormal and show increased interstitial markings, but the test of choice is a high-resolution CT of the chest. A lung biopsy is often necessary. In an initial evaluation, serology for rheumatoid factor (RF), antinuclear antibody (ANA), anti-Jo-1 antibody among others can be obtained.

Key Point
- ILD are a heterogeneous group of disorders that can be associated with exacerbations requiring a higher level of care.

4 Hemoptysis

Hemoptysis is the expectoration of blood from the respiratory tract.

4.1 General Considerations

Hemoptysis is uncommon and can be either massive or mild. Massive hemoptysis accounts for only approximately 10% of cases and is an emergency due to the possibility of rapid asphyxiation. Most cases of hemoptysis are mild and consist of blood-tinged sputum resulting from infections such as a viral bronchitis. Cavitary lesions from necrotizing pneumonia from *S. aureus* or *K. pneumoniae* and lung abscesses can cause hemoptysis. Cavitation from bronchogenic carcinoma can cause hemoptysis as can other pulmonary malignancies. Tuberculosis (TB) can also cause hemoptysis usually from cavitary lesions (see Chap. 2 on "Infectious Diseases"). Leptospirosis (see Chap. 2 on "Infectious Diseases") and mitral stenosis are rare but classic causes of hemoptysis. Pulmonary embolism (PE) can cause pulmonary infarction and production of hemoptysis (see Chap. 1 on "Cardiovascular Diseases"). Vasculitis such as granulomatosis with polyangiitis and Goodpasture's syndrome (pulmonary-renal syndromes) may cause hemoptysis. Diffuse alveolar hemorrhage (DAH) also known as idiopathic pulmonary hemorrhage (IPH) is a rare condition that can also present with hemoptysis. One of the most common causes of massive hemoptysis is from patients with bronchiectasis such as seen with cystic fibrosis and sarcoidosis.

4.2 History

Social and travel history should be taken. Massive hemoptysis can be defined as 150–200 mL at one time or 400 mL within 24 h. Patients may not be able to easily quantify an amount, but a U.S. cup (236 mL) can be used as a reference. Cough, fever, and shortness of breath may be reported in patients with pneumonia. Shortness of breath may also be reported in patients with PE and DAH. Patients with night sweats and weight loss may have TB.

4.3 Exam

Fever may be present with infection or PE. The pulse oximetry should be taken and documented. An examination of the nose and pharynx should be performed to check for a nasopharyngeal source of bleeding. The murmur of mitral stenosis may be present (opening snap with diastolic decrescendo murmur). Examination of the lungs may reveal adventitious sounds consistent with bronchitis or pneumonia. Lower extremity edema, usually unilateral, may be present with PE. Vasculitic rashes (see Chap. 13 on "Dermatology", Fig. 1) may be present with pulmonary-renal syndromes.

4.4 Diagnostics

A complete blood count can check for the anemia of blood loss that can occur with DAH. Testing for creatinine clearance will reveal renal failure seen with pulmonary-renal syndromes. A urinalysis can be performed in the office and will reveal hematuria in pulmonary-renal syndromes. A chest radiograph will be ordered in most patients with hemoptysis and can reveal pneumonia or TB. A CT will be ordered in smokers, patients greater than 40, and those suspected of PE.

Key Points
- Patients with massive hemoptysis should be referred to the ED.
- Hemoptysis is often associated with PE and TB which requires referral to the ED.
- Care should be taken in patients with bronchiectasis as these patients frequently have massive hemoptysis.

5 Pleural Effusion

Pleural effusion is an accumulation of fluid in the thorax between the visceral and parietal pleura.

5.1 General Considerations

Pleural effusions are fairly common, associated with common syndromes, and often are not a cause for an ED referral. The decision to refer the patient to the ED is primarily dependent on the proposed mechanism of production of the effusion or symptoms of the patient. Pleural effusions are classified as either transudative or exudative and this guides management in the hospital setting. Formerly, the light's criteria were devised to evaluate an effusion and were defined by a pleural effusion/serum protein ratio of 0.5 or greater or a pleural effusion/serum lactate dehydrogenase (LDH) ratio of 0.6 or greater. More recently a pleural fluid LDH more than 2/3 the upper limit of normal of the serum LDH or elevated pleural fluid cholesterol are used to evaluate an effusion. The most common cause of an effusion is congestive heart failure (CHF). CHF results in a transudative effusion. Another cause of a transudative effusion is hepatic hydrothorax which occurs in approximately 5% of patients with ascites. The most common cause of an exudative effusion is bacterial pneumonia. Viral pneumonias can also cause an exudative effusion and are probably responsible for a large number of "idiopathic" exudative effusions. A pulmonary embolism may cause an exudative effusion. The second most common cause of an exudative effusion is malignancy with carcinoma of lung and breast and lymphoma being the most common causes of a malignant effusion. A malignant effusion implies an advanced cancer and often care is palliative. Therefore, a malignant effusion cannot be missed and pleural effusions of unknown etiology must have a thoracentesis either in the hospital or done as an outpatient. Large effusions causing symptoms must also be admitted for drainage for relief and stabilization of the patient.

5.2 History

A history of CHF or cirrhosis may be elicited. The patient may relate a history of asbestosis. A recent abdominal surgery may be reported and can be an etiology for an exudative effusion. Sarcoidosis and collagen vascular diseases are another cause of exudative effusions. A fever may be reported with pneumonia. Shortness of breath and fatigue will often be the presenting symptoms. Chest pain may be reported with pneumonia, pulmonary embolism, and mesothelioma and these can be causes of exudative effusions.

5.3 Exam

The hallmark exam findings of a unilateral pleural effusion are unilateral decreased breath sounds and decreased tactile fremitus on the affected side. Tactile fremitus is assessed with the fingertips on the thorax while the patient is aerating the lungs by a prolonged pronunciation of the letter E. In contrast to a patient with a unilateral pleural effusion, a patient with a lobar infiltrate will have increased tactile fremitus on the affected side. Fever may be present with the parapneumonic effusion of a pneumonia. Pulse oximetry should be tested. Signs of congestive heart failure (CHF) such as jugular venous distention (JVD), an S3 heart sound, and lower extremity edema may be present (see Chap. 1 on "Cardiovascular Diseases"). Signs of ascites may be present such as abdominal distention and shifting dullness (see Chap. 3 on "Gastroenterology").

5.4 Diagnostics

A chest radiograph or chest CT can make the diagnosis. Cardiomegaly may be present with CHF.

Key Points
- Symptomatic pleural effusions are usually drained after admission to the hospital unless other mechanisms such as diuretics in CHF or paracentesis in cirrhosis with ascites can be utilized.

- Significant effusions of unknown etiology need to have a thoracentesis to evaluate for malignancy often in the hospital.

6 Pneumothorax

A pneumothorax is characterized by air filling the normally potential space between the visceral and parietal pleura.

6.1 General Considerations

A pneumothorax can be spontaneous (primary), secondary, iatrogenic, or traumatic. In the outpatient clinic, the most commonly seen will be a spontaneous pneumothorax due to a ruptured apical bleb in a smoker. The treatment for this is simple aspiration done in the ED. Secondary pneumothorax is most common in chronic obstructive pulmonary disease (COPD), though it can occur in any lung disease. Secondary pneumothorax is a more serious condition due to the decreased pulmonary reserve in these patients and is treated with a chest tube.

6.2 History

A history of smoking, infections, and trauma should be elicited. The classic finding is an acute onset of shortness of breath. Chest pain may be present.

6.3 Exam

The exam is variable. Classically, there are decreased breath sounds in a particular lung quadrant corresponding to the area of collapse, though this is not always found.

6.4 Diagnostics

A chest radiograph can be easily obtained and will show the classic lack of lung markings extending to the periphery of the chest wall.

Key Points
- Sudden onset of shortness of breath should be evaluated with a chest radiograph.
- A spontaneous pneumothorax is classically found in a thin young male smoker.

Further Reading

Cydulka RK, Fitch MT, Joing SA, Wang VJ, Cline DM, Ma OJ, editors. Tintinalli's emergency medicine manual. 8th ed. New York: McGraw Hill; 2018.

Jameson JL, Fauci AS, Kasper DL, Hauser SL, Longo DL, Loscalzo J, editors. Harrison's principles of internal medicine. 20th ed. New York: McGraw Hill; 2018.

Endocrinology

Gregory M. Booth

1 Introduction

The endocrine system is involved in the hormonal modulation of metabolism, energy production, and electrolytes that controls the global function of the human organism. Hormonal changes resulting in emergencies can be sudden or brought on gradually by the absence or decrease in hormonal amounts. The most common endocrine emergencies are caused by the ever-growing prevalence of diabetes in the USA in the form of diabetic ketoacidosis, hyperosmolar coma, and hypoglycemia. Emergencies involving the thyroid are not commonly encountered and the rare condition of acute suppurative thyroiditis is covered briefly. Hypoadrenalism is common, but adrenal crisis is rare in the absence of a previous diagnosis of adrenal insufficiency.

2 Diabetic Ketoacidosis

Diabetic ketoacidosis is a metabolic derangement that occurs in the absence or relative insufficiency of insulin.

G. M. Booth (✉)
Baltimore, MD, USA
e-mail: boothg444@yahoo.com

© The Author(s), under exclusive license to Springer Nature Switzerland AG 2022
G. M. Booth, S. Frattali (eds.), *Managing Emergencies in the Outpatient Setting*, https://doi.org/10.1007/978-3-031-15270-2_10

2.1 General Considerations

Admissions for diabetic ketoacidosis (DKA) are common and on the rise in the USA. DKA is most commonly seen in established type 1 diabetics who have stopped their insulin treatment, accidentally or through non-compliance. However, DKA can and does occur with relative frequency in type 2 diabetes. Additionally, DKA can be the initial presentation of diabetes in an ambulatory patient.

Criteria for a diagnosis of DKA include
- A blood glucose level greater than 250 mg/dL,
- The presence of serum ketones,
- An anion gap (AG) metabolic acidosis with an AG greater than 12,
- A serum bicarbonate less than 18 mEq/dL, and
- A pH less than 7.3

As such, DKA cannot be diagnosed definitively in the ambulatory setting. Euglycemic DKA is a recently discovered condition having the same parameters except a serum glucose less than 250 mg/dL, often seen with sodium glucose cotransporter-2 (SGLT-2) inhibitors. The pathophysiology of DKA is complex; it involves the production of an acidic hyperglycemic state through gluconeogenesis and lipolysis in the absence or relative insufficiency of insulin. The presence of the counterregulatory hormones glucagon, cortisol, growth hormone, and catecholamines also contribute to the hyperglycemia and acidosis. DKA often has precipitants such as myocardial infarction (MI), stroke, infection, and rarely, pregnancy. Medications such as corticosteroids, thiazide diuretics, and antipsychotics can precipitate DKA. Alcohol and illicit drug use often lead to non-compliance in diabetics on insulin. Alcohol can contribute to ketoacidosis and can also cause a separate entity, alcoholic ketoacidosis (AKA), not associated with DKA.

2.2 History

Patients in DKA often present with symptoms of sudden insulin absence, such as polydipsia and polyuria. The polyuria is often reported by patients to be more noticeable at night. Fatigue and weight loss is also common if the syndrome is subacute and accelerating. Gastrointestinal symptoms such as abdominal pain, nausea, and vomiting may be present. Patients may also have cognitive concerns.

2.3 Exam

Patients will often be dehydrated with tachycardia, hypotension, dry mucous membranes, and poor skin turgor. A fruity odor to the breath is also common due to the presence of ketones. The precipitants of DKA may be present as seen in MI (see

Chap. 1 "Cardiology Diseases"), stroke (see Chap. 4 "Neurology"), and infections (see Chap. 2 on "Infectious Disease").

2.4 Diagnostics

The blood glucose seen on glucometer is usually but not always greater than 250 mg/dL. Lower glucose values can be seen often in those patients on SGLT-2 inhibitors. The urinalysis will show ketones, a sensitive (98%) but not specific (35%) finding in DKA. In the appropriate setting, an EKG should be obtained in patients who are suspected of DKA and cardiac issues.

Key Points
- DKA is a potentially fatal condition in both type 1 and 2 diabetics and can be the initial presentation of diabetes.
- In symptomatic patients with a glucose greater than 250 mg/dL and significant ketones on urinalysis, an ED referral is required to rule out the presence of DKA.

3 Hyperglycemic Hyperosmolar State

Hyperglycemic hyperosmolar state (HHS) is characterized by hyperglycemia and a highly concentrated serum.

3.1 General Considerations

HHS is related to DKA in that both have an elevated glucose level and marked electrolyte disturbance, but HHS lacks the typical acidosis associated with DKA. HHS is typically found in type 2 diabetics. In HHS, glucose is often markedly increased at 600 mg/dL and above, and the patient's mental status is often altered. DKA often presents more acutely, especially in established type 1 diabetics, but HHS may present subacutely over days to weeks. Like DKA, a careful history on precipitants such as infection and cardiovascular disorders should be taken.

3.2 History

Polyuria, polydipsia, and weight loss may be reported. Blurry vision and altered mental status are also common. Gastrointestinal symptoms, however, are not as prominent as in DKA.

3.3 Exam

Hypotension or orthostasis may be present due to dehydration. Tachycardia, dry mucous membranes and poor skin turgor are other signs of dehydration. The patient may also possess an altered mental status ranging from mild to profound. Focal neurologic signs may be present.

3.4 Diagnostics

The fingerstick in the office will often not register the value, but if present will be around 600 mg/dL or above. The basic metabolic panel will show an elevated BUN, creatinine, and serum osmolality greater than 320 mOsmol.

Key Points
- Patients with altered mental status and/or dehydration may have elevations in glucose and hyperglycemic hyperosmolar state.
- HHS will often have glucose values above 600 mg/dL (or be unregistrable) by glucometer in the clinic.

4 Hypoglycemia

4.1 General Considerations

Hypoglycemia is extremely common in the diabetic population, especially those on insulin or sulfonylureas. No specific level of blood sugar can be used to define hypoglycemia; however, hypoglycemia is commonly defined as a glucose of less than 70 mg/dL. At this level, brain glucose uptake is reduced, and symptoms begin to develop. At around 60 mg/dL autonomic symptoms begin to develop, and they include hunger, anxiety, palpitations, tremor, sweating, and nausea. When the levels drop below 50 mg/dL, neuroglycopenic symptoms such as blurry vision and dizziness occur. Sometimes more serious symptoms develop at this level such as slurred speech and confusion. Seizures, progression of confusion, obtundation, and permanent neurologic deficits can ensue if the glucose levels fall below this level. The most common cause of hypoglycemia is the skipping of meals by diabetic patients on hypoglycemic drugs such as sulfonylureas or insulin. A sudden decline in renal function can also lead to hypoglycemia in patients on these drugs. Other causes apart from diabetes can cause hypoglycemia. Alcohol use and liver impairment can cause hypoglycemia, and patients with these comorbidities should be closely monitored. Hypoglycemia can also be associated with dumping syndrome in bariatric surgery patients. Rarer causes of hypoglycemia include adrenal insufficiency, insulinoma, and insulin autoimmunity. In situations of abuse of diabetic medications, levels of sulfonylureas can be measured. The discussion of a more complex evaluation of hypoglycemia is beyond the scope of this book.

4.2 Treatment

Often, hypoglycemia is managed based on a protocol approved by the medical director/physician in the practice. An example would be, when hypoglycemia (50–60 mg/dL) is confronted in the clinic or by telephone call, patients should be administered 15 g of carbohydrates such as 4 oz of fruit juice or regular soda. After 15 min, the finger stick should be checked again and, if the patient is still hypoglycemic, another 15 g should be administered. If the patient is still significantly hypoglycemic after another 15 min, EMS should be activated. If the glucose level does respond, 15–20 g of complex carbohydrate such as bread or crackers should be given. If a patient has severe neuroglycopenic symptoms, then EMS should be called immediately.

4.3 Diagnostics

Glucometer values (less than 70) should be used for diagnosis. (Point of care A1C can also be useful to indicate persistently low glucose values, if it is available). Introductory laboratory investigations of persistent hypoglycemia also include kidney and liver function tests. Simultaneous evaluation of glucose, insulin, c-peptide, and sulfonylureas can also be ordered as an outpatient for a more complete analysis.

Key Points
- Patients with significant neuroglycopenic symptoms on hypoglycemic medications need immediate monitoring and IV glucose with EMS transport.
- If hypoglycemia does not respond to two administrations of 15 g of simple carbohydrates 15 min apart, then EMS should be activated.

5 Thyroid Storm

Severe thyrotoxicosis, or thyroid storm, is a rare syndrome affecting multiple organ systems caused by overproduction of thyroid hormone.

5.1 General Considerations

Thyroid storm is an extremely rare condition. Thyroid storm is the term for life-threatening severe thyrotoxicosis that needs immediate identification and treatment. Identifying patients with thyroid storm is often not clear; however, the Burch–Wartofsky diagnostic criteria have been developed to aid evaluation. These criteria produce a numbered score denoting the likely, impending, and unlikely presence of thyroid storm. The criteria are composed of vital signs (temperature and pulse), cardiovascular system dysfunction (congestive heart failure), central nervous system dysfunction, and gastro-hepatic symptoms and signs. One criterion is the presence of a precipitant, which can include infections, coronary syndromes, pulmonary embolism, trauma, surgery, childbirth, and discontinuation of treatment for hyperthyroidism. Often, no precipitant is found, and the diagnosis is derived from a new case of Graves disease, toxic multinodular goiter, various neoplasms (pituitary, trophoblastic tumor, choriocarcinoma, ovarian teratoma), and hyperemesis gravidarum. Another mechanism is release of preformed thyroid hormone from infections of the thyroid gland, medication reactions (amiodarone), post-partum and sporadic thyroiditis, and surgical manipulation.

5.2 History

A history of thyroid abnormalities is common but not always present. Pain in the neck around the area of the thyroid gland (found in infections and inflammation) can also be reported. Cardiovascular symptoms such as palpitations and shortness of breath may be reported or chest pain with an acute coronary syndrome as a precipitant. Neurological symptoms such as confusion and lethargy can occur especially in the elderly. Symptoms more specific to hyperthyroidism are weight loss, heat intolerance, and muscle weakness. Gastrointestinal symptoms such as nausea, vomiting, and diarrhea are also possible symptoms.

5.3 Exam

Temperature and pulse are often elevated. An irregularly irregular pulse is associated with atrial fibrillation, if present. Signs of congestive heart failure such as an S3 sound, jugular venous distension, lung rales, and lower extremity edema may be seen. Jaundice from congestive hepatopathy may be present. Signs more specific to thyrotoxicosis are the neurological findings of a tremor and hyperreflexia and an enlarged and/or tender thyroid gland. A thyroid bruit is pathognomonic for Grave's disease.

5.4 Diagnostics

The diagnostic finding will be an undetectable TSH. A CBC may have an elevated white count indicating an infection as a precipitant. The bilirubin may be elevated in jaundice. The EKG may reveal atrial fibrillation or the findings of an acute coronary syndrome. A chest radiograph may reveal congestive heart failure.

Key Points
- Patients with findings consistent with thyroid storm should be hospitalized for treatment considering the mortality associated with this condition.
- Commonly, though not always, there will be precipitants of thyroid storm.

6 Myxedema

Myxedema is a profound hypothyroidism affecting various body systems with a potentially fatal outcome.

6.1 General Considerations

Myxedema is an extremely rare condition that usually occurs in patients with a pre-existing diagnosis of hypothyroidism. The most common underlying condition is Hashimoto's thyroiditis, but other conditions such as thyroidectomy, radioactive iodine, and medications such as lithium and amiodarone may also be causative. Decompensation from various factors may play a role. Infections, congestive heart failure, metabolic disturbances, and drugs, especially sedatives and narcotics are all factors that may be present in an outpatient setting.

6.2 History

A history of hypothyroidism is almost always present, but an altered patient may not relate this historical fact. Patients who are comatose will not be evaluated in the outpatient setting; however, more subtle presentations have occurred. Examples include depression, paranoia, or hallucinations. GI symptoms such as anorexia, abdominal pain, and constipation may be reported. Myxedema affects multiple systems that are evaluated on exam.

6.3 Exam

The vital signs may reveal hypothermia and bradycardia. Hypotension may be present. The patient may also be lethargic or altered. A harsh voice may be present due to edema in the vocal cords. Macroglossia may occur as part of the generalized edema. Upon further examination, the patient may possess a scar from a previous thyroidectomy. Decreased heart sounds from a pericardial effusion may be present. A generalized edematous state may also be present with pulmonary edema and lower extremity edema. As with less profound presentations of hypothyroidism, a lack of body hair and dry scaly skin may be present. Bruising may be present on the skin due to the coagulopathy associated with severe hypothyroidism. Deep tendon reflexes are decreased or absent.

6.4 Diagnostics

Anemia from several mechanisms may be present. Hyponatremia, hypoglycemia, and hypercalcemia are commonly encountered metabolic derangements. The EKG may have multiple abnormalities. Bradycardia and a prolonged QT interval may be present. If a pericardial effusion is present, low voltage and inverted T-waves may be reported.

Key Point
- Altered mental status or psychiatric abnormalities in the presence of an abnormal examination consistent with severe hypothyroidism is a precursor to decompensation leading to myxedema. These patients should be referred to the ED.

7 Adrenal Crisis

Adrenal crisis is caused by a sudden lack of sufficient cortisol in the serum resulting in circulatory collapse.

7.1 General Considerations

Adrenal crisis can occur spontaneously in patients who do not carry a diagnosis of adrenal insufficiency or in patients with the diagnosis of adrenal insufficiency (AI) who encounter increased needs for cortisol in response to infection, injury, trauma, or major surgery. Forty percent of patients with chronic AI have encountered a crisis in their lifetime, and 20% of patients will experience more than one crisis in their lifetime. Adrenal crises are therefore quite common. AI can be primary (in the adrenal glands) or secondary (in the pituitary).

The list of causes of primary AI is quite long and includes
- Autoimmune (Addison's disease)
- Neoplastic (usually from metastasis)
- Infectious causes (classically tuberculosis)
- Infiltrative (hemochromatosis and amyloidosis)
- Drug induced causes (such as ketoconazole and opioids)
- Hemorrhage

Secondary causes of AI are
- Glucocorticoids (most common)
- Immune checkpoint inhibitors
- Hemorrhage

Hemorrhage can occur into the adrenals or pituitary. It can occur spontaneously in those on anticoagulants or those with antiphospholipid antibody syndrome. Hemorrhage into the pituitary can also occur in the post-partum state especially in cases of prolonged hypotension (Sheehan's syndrome—Sect. 8). Hemorrhage into the adrenal gland can occur with infections called Waterhouse–Friderichsen syndrome—classically seen with meningococcus. Immune checkpoint inhibitors (CTLA-4 inhibitors, PD-1 inhibitors, and PDL-1 inhibitors) are a special case as they cause hypophysitis (inflammation of the pituitary) and often cause pituitary dysfunction in more than one domain.

7.2 History

Chronic AI is associated with vague symptoms that include fatigue, weight loss, myalgias and arthralgias. Gastrointestinal symptoms such as anorexia, nausea, vomiting, and diarrhea can also occur. Adrenal crisis is suggested by confusion, severe weakness, acute abdominal pain, and history of fevers and syncope. Acute headache may be present in those with pituitary apoplexy (see below).

7.3 Exam

Fever may be present. Hypotension can occur which may begin as orthostatic hypotension in chronic AI. Fever and hypotension are often interpreted as sepsis in an adrenal crisis, and they can present simultaneously (Waterhouse–Friderichsen syndrome). Abdominal pain and guarding may be present and can be confused with an acute abdomen. Skin findings may be present such as vitiligo (classic with Addison's disease) or hyperpigmentation seen in chronic primary AI.

7.4 Diagnostics

The basic metabolic panel classically shows hyponatremia in both primary and secondary AI, and hyperkalemia also can occur in primary AI due to the absence of mineralocorticoids. Hypoglycemia can occur in adrenal crisis (less commonly in primary AI) and can be assessed in the office with a glucometer. Hypercalcemia can also occur in both chronic and acute AI. If acute adrenal hemorrhage is suspected, a CT scan can be ordered and will reveal the typical abnormalities associated with this syndrome.

Key Points
- Adrenal crisis can occur in those with previous diagnosis of chronic AI and requires circulatory support in the hospital.
- In patients with hypotension of unknown etiology, a high index of suspicion must be maintained for the syndromic factors associated with an adrenal crisis.
- Metabolic abnormalities seen on the basic metabolic panel include hyponatremia (most common), hyperkalemia (primary AI only), hypoglycemia, and hypercalcemia.

8 Pituitary Apoplexy

Pituitary apoplexy is an infarction or hemorrhage of the pituitary that produces stroke-like symptoms and a characteristic clinical syndrome.

8.1 General Considerations

Pituitary apoplexy is extremely rare with approximately 500 cases per year in the USA. The syndrome affects both sexes equally and most commonly occurs in the 5–6th decade of life. Not all cases are sudden; the onset may be subtle and subacute, manifesting over days to months. Most often, pituitary apoplexy develops from an existing pituitary macroadenoma. The larger the size of the adenoma the more likely the onset of pituitary apoplexy. With that said, microadenomas can apoplex. In the majority of cases there is no clear precipitant; however, patients on anticoagulation are at increased risk. A classic cause of pituitary apoplexy is the post-partum state after an episode of hypotension (Sheehan's syndrome). Hypertension and sharp fluctuations in blood pressure are common precipitants of hemorrhagic infarcts (see Chap. 4 "Neurology"). Pituitary apoplexy can also occur as a result of surgeries due to hypotensive episodes (as in cardiopulmonary bypass) or microemboli from vascular procedures in those patients with atherosclerosis (rare). The symptoms are generally similar to a hemorrhagic stroke with an additional sudden onset of hypopituitarism.

8.2 History

The typical history of pituitary apoplexy is a sudden onset of headache and altered mental status, though altered mental status is present only 3–19% of the time. A stiff neck may be reported. Photophobia and nausea and vomiting are often present as in other hemorrhagic strokes. Visual disturbances are often reported either acutely or in a progressive fashion. In more subacute cases, fatigue and the dysfunction typically associated with the sex and thyroid hormones can be reported.

8.3 Exam

The patient may be hypotensive due to the abrupt onset of adrenal insufficiency. Pupillary responses are affected approximately 20% of the time. Visual acuity loss and visual field abnormalities are present approximately 20–50% of the time. Ocular palsies are common. More significant neurologic deficits can be possible depending on the extent of the infarction.

8.4 Diagnostics

The basic metabolic panel will show the hyponatremia of secondary adrenal insufficiency. An 8 a.m. cortisol often may be less than 3.0 g/dL. Central hypothyroidism (a low TSH and T4) and central hypogonadism (low LH and FSH with a low estrogen and testosterone) may be present. A CT can be useful, often showing hemorrhage and a pituitary mass; however, MRI is the imaging test of choice.

Key Points
- Pituitary apoplexy is characterized by the findings of a hemorrhagic stroke and pituitary abnormalities.
- Subacute presentations are possible.
- A CT is easy to get and may show the abnormality, but an MRI with pituitary protocol is the imaging test of choice.

9 Hypercalcemia

Hypercalcemia is an overabundance of the calcium ion in the bloodstream.

9.1 General Considerations

Severe hypercalcemia is caused by two mechanisms in 90% of cases and they are via parathyroid hormone (PTH)-related mechanisms (primary hyperparathyroidism) and hypercalcemia of malignancy (HOM). Most cases of HOM are found in patients with a known malignancy (solid tumors and lymphoma) and portend a poor prognosis. Other causes of hypercalcemia are end stage renal disease (see Chap. 5 on "Nephrology"), thiazide diuretics, lithium, and overuse of supplements such as vitamin D and calcium containing compounds (i.e., antacids). Several rare genetic disorders such as multiple endocrine neoplasia (MEN 1 and MEN2A) and familial hypocalciuric hypercalcemia are also on the differential. Most cases of severe hypercalcemia are found in cancer patients and as a "parathyroid" crisis associated with primary hyperparathyroidism. The rapidity of onset plays a role in the body's response to hypercalcemia in addition to the absolute numerical value of the calcium level. The treatment for hypercalcemia is aggressive fluid administration and bisphosphonates. Furosemide, calcitonin, and denosumab (instead of bisphosphonates) are also used in select cases.

9.2 History

Symptoms of hypercalcemia can be associated with their effects on the body's metabolism. Polydipsia and polyuria are common and can cause dehydration, which in turn can cause headaches, weakness, and syncope/presyncope. Abdominal pain due to constipation and neural stimulation is common. Psychiatric symptoms, lethargy, and even altered mental status are possible. Current or historical symptoms of kidney stones can be elicited.

9.3 Exam

Hypotension due to dehydration occurs frequently. Abdominal tenderness can be present. Subtle signs of altered cognition may also be present.

9.4 Diagnostics

The first step in the evaluation of hypercalcemia is to correct the value for the presence of hypoalbuminemia if necessary. The calcium value should be reduced 0.8 mg/dL for every 1.0 g/dL decrease in serum albumin. Most cases of severe hypercalcemia (14.0 mg/dL or more) should be referred to the hospital. Moderate cases of hypercalcemia (12–14 mg/dL) should be evaluated based on the severity of symptoms.

Key Points
- In patients with a history of cancer or primary hyperparathyroidism, symptoms consistent with severe hypercalcemia should be referred to the hospital.
- A patient with a calcium level of 14.0 mg/dL or more should be referred to the ED.
- Moderate hypercalcemia (12–14 mg/dL) should be managed based on fluid status.

10 Hypocalcemia

Hypocalcemia is a low level of the calcium ion in the cardiovascular system.

10.1 General Considerations

Hypocalcemic crisis is caused by a lack of parathyroid hormone caused by surgery to the parathyroid and thyroid glands. Parathyroid surgery for primary hyperparathyroidism is associated with hypocalcemia approximately 1–2% of the time and is typically transient. Prolonged hypocalcemia can be caused by "hungry bones syndrome," seen with previous hypoparathyroid bone disease, and can last for days to months. Thyroid surgery is a more common procedure and frequently the cause of transient or permanent hypoparathyroidism, which is a complication seen between 0.5 and 5% of the time. Risk factors for postoperative hypoparathyroidism are Grave's disease, Hashimoto's thyroiditis, bilateral neck dissection, and surgery for malignancy. Hypomagnesemia is associated with suppression of the parathyroid gland and hypocalcemia. Levels of this cation should always be checked and repleted in cases of hypocalcemia. The level of hypocalcemia resulting in the need for IV supplementation depends on symptoms; however, levels below 7.0 g/dL are concerning. Early symptoms such as circumoral tingling, twitching, and paresthesias should be rapidly treated.

10.2 History

The history of previous recent surgery to the thyroid or parathyroid is usually elicited. The symptoms of hypocalcemia are caused by the neuromuscular excitability of the sensory and motor nerves caused by a lowering of the threshold for neuron firing. Symptoms can range from paresthesias, numbness, and muscle spasms to tetany, bronchospasm, laryngospasm, and arrhythmias. Cognitive and psychiatric symptoms such as confusion, anxiety, and irritability may also occur.

10.3 Physical Exam

Bradycardia may be present. Two common exam findings besides obvious twitching and tetany are Chvostek's sign and Trousseau's sign. Chvostek's sign is facial spasm induced by tapping of the facial nerve 2 cm anterior to the auditory canal. Trousseau's sign is carpal spasm with inflation of a blood pressure cuff slightly above systolic pressure for 2–3 min. Chvostek's sign is a normal finding in 10% of patients but Trousseau's sign is much more specific.

10.4 Diagnostics

The metabolic panel will reveal a low calcium below 8.0 g/dL. A magnesium should always be checked and replaced if low. A vitamin D level should be measured. An EKG will reveal a prolonged QT interval which can be associated with ventricular arrhythmias.

Key Points
- Symptomatic hypocalcemia is concerning and associated with significant morbidity and mortality.
- Chvostek and Trousseau's signs can help diagnose hypocalcemia clinically.
- Levels below 7.0 should raise concern for the need of IV replacement especially if associated with symptoms.

11 Acute Suppurative Thyroiditis

Acute suppurative thyroiditis is a rare potentially life-threatening infection of the thyroid gland.

11.1 General Considerations

Acute suppurative thyroiditis (AST) is an extremely rare condition with most of the literature reported as case series. Infection of the thyroid gland is rare due to the natural defenses of high iodine content, extensive vascularity and lymphatic drainage, and encapsulation. Predisposing factors for AST include immunosuppression, the presence of a pyriform sinus fistula, neck trauma, previous fine needle aspiration (FNA), or from contiguous or hematogenous spread. Most AST is due to bacterial infection such as *Staphylococcus* and *Streptococcus* species but gram-negative infection is also possible as is fungal and mycobacterial causes. The diagnosis is often difficult to differentiate from the non-emergent diagnosis of subacute painful thyroiditis which often causes pain and thyrotoxicosis. Prednisone is sometimes used with subacute painful thyroiditis; however, it should be administered with caution. If a misdiagnosis is made, and the condition is actually AST, prednisone can cause a worsening of this serious infection.

11.2 History

The physician should inquire about predisposing factors such as an immunocompromised state and history of FNA. Symptoms of infections such as fever and neck pain may be reported. Symptoms of thyrotoxicosis are as previously delineated (see above). Symptoms of hyperthyroidism are weight loss, heat intolerance, and muscle weakness. Gastrointestinal symptoms such as nausea, vomiting and diarrhea may be present.

11.3 Exam

Fever may be present. Signs specific to the thyroid gland may be present such as thyroid tenderness, redness, and swelling. Signs of thyrotoxicosis such as tachycardia, tremor, and hyperreflexia may be present. These are not specific to AST as subacute painful thyroiditis may also cause these signs.

11.4 Diagnostics

A white count with a CBC and elevations of ESR and CRP may be present. These are not specific to AST as they are also found with the non-emergent entity subacute painful thyroiditis. An ultrasound is more sensitive than CT in the early stages of AST, though a CT is nearly 100% sensitive in the acute symptomatic stages of AST.

Key Points
- Acute suppurative thyroiditis is a rare life-threatening infection of the thyroid gland that is associated with pain, redness, and swelling of the gland.
- An ultrasound is more sensitive early in the disease process than a CT.
- When signs of hyperthyroidism are present, the CT is the test of choice.

Further Reading

Cydulka RK, Fitch MT, Joing SA, Wang VJ, Cline DM, Ma J, editors. Tintinalli's emergency medicine manual. 8th ed. New York: McGraw Hill; 2018.
Shifrin AL. Endocrine emergencies. Amsterdam: Elsevier; 2022.

Hematology and Oncology

Gregory M. Booth

1 Introduction

Referrals to the emergency department (ED) as it relates to hematology and oncology can be based on the clinical scenario or results of the complete blood count (CBC). Cases of spinal cord compression and acute leukemia often can be sent to the ED on clinical grounds without imaging or laboratory testing. Other times, abnormalities on the CBC prompt ED referral when results are reported after the patient's visit. Hyperviscosity syndrome, severe symptomatic anemia, and severe thrombocytopenia are covered in this chapter. Neutropenic fever is covered in the Chapter on "Infectious Diseases". Hemophilia and sickle cell disease are genetic hematologic disorders that have certain indications for an ED referral.

2 Spinal Cord Compression

Spinal cord compression is an external pressure on the spinal cord that is usually from an external metastatic malignancy compressing on the surrounding tissues.

G. M. Booth (✉)
Baltimore, MD, USA
e-mail: boothg444@yahoo.com

2.1 General Considerations

Lung, breast, and prostate cancer are the neoplasms mostly likely to metastasize to the spine, accounting for 60% of cases. Renal cell carcinoma, non-Hodgkin's lymphoma, and multiple myeloma each account for 5–10% of cases. The remainder of cases are from colorectal cancer, primary of unknown origin, and sarcoma. In 20% of these patients, spinal cord compression is the presenting condition, and one-third of these patients have lung cancer. Spinal cord compression is a grave condition; most patients survive for only 3–6 months after diagnosis. However, prompt recognition and treatment of spinal cord compression can avoid considerable morbidity and preserve ambulatory status and quality of life.

2.2 History

Back pain is the presenting symptom in 90% of cases. In spinal cord compression, the aching or gnawing pain increases in the supine position and with the Valsalva maneuver. The thoracic region is commonly affected in cord compression. Symptoms in this region should cause concern for secondary back pain as mechanical causes of back pain are less common in this region. Patients commonly describe band paresthesia around the thoracic region as "squeezed like a belt being pulled tight" or a "band of numbness around the waist."

2.3 Exam

Palpation over the vertebrae can elicit pain from metastatic deposits. Signs of neurologic compromise such as muscle weakness is an ominous sign and should prompt an emergent response. Leg ataxia may precede weakness, and the gait of the patient should be examined. Hyperreflexia may be present and the Babinski sign should be performed. If movement of the great toe is equivocal, then movement of the four lateral toes should be examined with stimulation of the lateral aspect of the foot. Movement of the four lateral toes is often a more reliable finding. Anal sphincter tone should be assessed; if the patient is immunosuppressed, a gloved finger adjacent to (not in) the canal can be used during attempted activation of the sphincter.

2.4 Diagnostics

Inflammatory markers (SED rate and CRP) can be used to evaluate for abscess if this is in the differential diagnosis (see Chap. 4 on "Neurology"). An MRI is about 95% sensitive and specific to cord compression and should be ordered for the thoracic and lumbar spine. In general, an X-ray should not be ordered as significant bone loss is necessary to generate a positive exam.

Key Points
- Back pain in patients with cancer should generally prompt swift imaging.
- Spinal cord compression is the presenting symptom in 20% of these patients and the thoracic spine is a common location.
- Hyperreflexia and neuromuscular compromise should be assessed immediately and used to make treatment decisions to preserve ambulatory function.
- An MRI is about 95% sensitive and specific to cord compression.

3 Acute Leukemia

Leukemia is an uncontrolled proliferation of blood cell progenitors resulting in widespread organ dysfunction.

3.1 General Considerations

The most common acute leukemia in adults is acute myeloid leukemia (AML) with approximately 20,000 cases occurring annually. The median age at diagnosis is 67 years of age. The prognosis for AML is grim, with a 27% chance of survival at 5 years. Most cases of AML are sporadic, with genetic predisposition in those individuals with Down syndrome, Fanconi anemia, ataxia-telangiectasia, and other rare conditions. AML can also occur following therapy for other cancers such as with alkylating agents, topoisomerase II inhibitors, or ionizing radiation. AML can also occur with transformations from chronic myelogenous leukemia (CML) and chronic lymphocytic leukemia (CLL). Acute lymphocytic leukemia is rarely seen in adults. In some populations, it is associated with the human T-lymphotropic virus-1 (HTLV-1) virus in adults.

3.2 History

The most common initial symptom with AML is fatigue. The patient also may report fevers, anorexia, and weight loss. Effects on hemostasis, such as mucosal bleeding and easy bruising, can also be reported. Expansion of the bone marrow with infiltrative cells may result in diffuse "bone pain." The patient may report a lump that is from AML (see below). Symptoms of various infections affecting various body systems—skin, lung etc. may be present. Some subtypes of leukemia have catastrophic bleeding, including intracranial hemorrhage (ICH). Therefore, symptoms of a headache should not be ignored in this context.

3.3 Exam

Fever may be present. Signs of infection such as cellulitis, pneumonia, etc. may be present (see Chap. 2 on "Infectious Emergencies"). Bruising may be apparent. Hepatosplenomegaly may be found, although it is not common. A myeloid sarcoma, a mass of myeloid cells, can be found in the skin and the testis on rare occasions as well.

3.4 Diagnostic Tests

A decreased hemoglobin may be present on the complete blood count (CBC) but may not be severe. Platelet counts less than 100,000 cells per microliter (μL) are found 75% of the time. The CBC counts of the leukocytes can vary, with a median count of 15,000 cells per μL. Between 25 and 40% have low counts, and 20% have counts greater than 100,000. Over 95% of patients have blasts in the peripheral blood.

Key Point
- Patients suspected of acute leukemia based on their symptoms, signs, and CBC should be referred to the ED or for prompt hematology-oncology referral depending on their presentation and blood counts.

4 Hyperviscosity Syndrome

Hyperviscosity syndrome (HVS) is an emergency caused by increased levels of blood components or immunoglobulins.

4.1 General Considerations

Hyperviscosity syndrome (HVS) is most commonly seen in diseases such as Waldenstrom's macroglobulinemia and multiple myeloma resulting from increased levels of immunoglobulins, especially IgM. HVS can also occur from large increases in red blood cells in polycythemia vera cases, platelets in thrombocytosis cases, and white blood cells (WBC) in leukemia cases. Increased serum viscosity causes ischemia in the capillaries of various organs causing a myriad of different clinical manifestations the most important being in the neurologic and cardiovascular systems. Leukostasis is defined as symptomatic hyperleukocytosis with a WBC count greater than 100,000 cells per μL. This is most commonly associated with acute myeloid leukemia (AML), but can also occur with acute lymphocytic leukemia (ALL) and chronic myeloid leukemia (CML). Rarely, thrombocytosis can occur with active thrombosis and requires emergent therapy.

4.2 History

A fever may be present if the patient has a concurrent infection. The patient will likely have a current cancer diagnosis but not always. Approximately, 10–20% of AML patients present with leukostasis. Involvement of the pulmonary system will result in shortness of breath and dyspnea on exertion which can progress to acute respiratory distress syndrome. Neurologic symptoms include headaches, vision changes, and dizziness.

4.3 Exam

Fever and hypertension may be present. Signs of heart failure may be present including crackles in the lungs. The neurologic exam may be abnormal, especially ataxia and cognitive changes.

4.4 Diagnostics

The complete blood count will be markedly abnormal as described above with possible increases in erythrocytes, leukocytes, and platelets. The metabolic panel may reveal renal failure and electrolyte abnormalities.

Key Points
- Symptomatic, dramatic elevations in leukocytes, erythrocytes, or platelets require emergent care.
- The cardiovascular and neurologic systems are the most commonly affected systems.
- New pulmonary or neurologic symptoms in patients with Waldenstrom's macroglobulinemia or multiple myeloma should prompt consideration for prompt hematology referral, in the ED if necessary.

5 Anemia

Anemia is characterized by a low hemoglobin and hematocrit and arises from a variety of etiologies.

5.1 General Considerations

The etiology of anemia is beyond the scope of this section; however, some basic parameters will be briefly discussed. In the outpatient setting, the complete blood count (CBC) will be interpreted in retrospect after the office visit. The first aspect of the CBC to consider is the degree of the anemia. Generally, a hemoglobin less than 7 or hematocrit less than 21 is considered an emergency requiring ED referral for transfusion. Higher levels of hemoglobin can be considered for ED referral if the patient is likely to be dehydrated or is symptomatic. The patient's underlying conditions are also a consideration as cardiac patients and patients with leukemia require a higher hemoglobin level due to their higher oxygen requirements. The mean corpuscular volume (MCV) is the first determinant of the approach to anemia. A low MCV (microcytic anemia) is the most common finding in outpatients with severe anemia and implies chronic blood loss often from the GI tract. Often these patients are without complaint, but on further questioning, are usually symptomatic with fatigue. These patients are often admitted to expedite their work-up and get transfusion of blood products. A rare cause is that of microangiopathic hemolytic anemia which has a low platelet count in addition to anemia (see Chap. 5 "Nephrology"). It should be noted cirrhosis can also cause a low platelet count due to splenic sequestration (see Chap. 3 on "Gastro Enterology"). Use of alcohol or liver disease may increase the MCV and hide a predominantly microcytic picture of anemia.

5.2 History

A history of consumption of NSAIDs is a risk for peptic ulcer disease which may be asymptomatic or minimally symptomatic with nausea and dyspepsia. A history of fatigue is usually present. Shortness of breath with minimal or less than normal exertion can be reported especially in the older population. A history of dark-colored stools (melena) from an intestinal bleed should be elicited.

5.3 Exam

Pallor of the skin, nail beds, and conjunctiva may be appreciated. Tachycardia and hypotension may be a compensatory mechanism found later in the disease course.

5.4 Diagnostics

If a high suspicion for severe anemia is present, a spun hematocrit is sometimes available in the clinic and a hematocrit of less than 21 is a definite criterion for admission for transfusion.

Key Points
- In most cases, a hemoglobin of 7 or less should be referred to the ED for evaluation and likely transfusion of blood products.
- Patients who are symptomatic or with cardiac disease or leukemia may have a higher threshold for transfusion.
- Dehydrated patients will have hemoconcentration, and their hemoglobin will decrease with administration of IV fluids.

6 Thrombocytopenia

Thrombocytopenia is the drop in platelets beyond the commonly accepted threshold of 150,000 per microliter (μL).

6.1 General Considerations

Thrombocytopenia is common and generally not thought to be attributable to bleeding until the level reaches less than 50,000 cells per microliter (μL). This is a generalization and the effect on bleeding depends on platelet function and other pathophysiologic mechanisms. Bleeding can range from minor and superficial such as mucosal bleeding to life-threatening intracranial hemorrhage. The actual cause may be due to decreased marrow production or increased peripheral destruction. The differential for thrombocytopenia in the previously healthy patient is long with autoimmune, malignant, medication reaction, and viral etiologies as the common culprits. Another common cause is splenic sequestration from various etiologies such as leukemia or cirrhosis. In a healthy, asymptomatic patient, the most common cause is increased destruction due to autoimmune mechanisms referred to as ITP (immune thrombocytopenic purpura or idiopathic thrombocytopenic purpura). In patients with likely ITP, platelet levels above 30,000 cells per μL have been found to not affect mortality. Heparin-induced-thrombocytopenia (HIT) and thrombotic thrombocytopenic purpura (TTP) are two diseases that combine thrombocytopenia with thrombosis. HIT can occur 5–14 days after initiation of heparin including low-molecular-weight heparins (LMWHs) such as enoxaparin. HIT can rarely develop several days after heparin has been stopped. This is termed delayed onset HIT. HIT requires a prompt hematologic evaluation. Thrombotic thrombocytopenic purpura is another rare cause of thrombocytopenia associated with thrombosis that has been described elsewhere in this book (see Chap. 5 on "Nephrology").

6.2 History

The medications of the patient must be carefully reviewed as the list of drugs commonly associated with thrombocytopenia is quite long. This includes very common over-the-counter medications such as acetaminophen and naproxen, and antibiotics such as beta-lactams. The patient may report a history of mucosal bleeding during dental care. Bruising may be reported which should be apparent on exam. More serious symptoms such as gastrointestinal bleeding (see Chap. 3 on "Gastroenterology") and headaches from intracranial hemorrhage (see Chap. 4 on "Neurology") may be apparent.

6.3 Exam

Bruising appears due to either decreased platelet number or function. Petechiae, pin-point non-blanching hemorrhages that denote decreased platelet number not function, may also be present. Purpuric, "wet" blisters on the oral mucosa are indicative of potential catastrophic bleeding and should be referred for immediate evaluation. The spleen should be evaluated in the thrombocytopenic patient and may be found to be enlarged.

6.4 Diagnostics

The laboratory evaluation of thrombocytopenia in a non-critical patient includes testing for platelet clumping with a peripheral smear and retesting in a tube without ethylenediamine tetraacetic acid (EDTA). The presence of anemia may indicate TTP. If splenomegaly needs to be evaluated, an abdominal ultrasound or CT scan can be ordered.

Key Points
- "Wet" purpura in the oral mucosa has been associated with catastrophic bleeding and should be evaluated in the ED.
- Thrombocytopenia associated with bleeding should be monitored in the ED.
- Bleeding does not usually occur until the platelet count drops below 30,000 cells per µL, and these patients should have repeat blood work drawn immediately in the ED.
- Patients with platelet counts found to be less than 20,000 cells per µL should be referred for hospitalization.

7 Hemarthrosis and Hemophilia

Hemarthrosis is the infiltration of blood products into the joint space and is a common sequela of hemophilia.

7.1 General Considerations

Hemarthrosis generally occurs in the setting of hemophilia (85%), although cases with anticoagulation, thrombocytopenia, von Willebrand disease, or factor V deficiency do occur. Hemophilia is a sex-linked recessive disease caused by the absence or deficiency of factor VIII (hemophilia A or classic hemophilia) or factor IX (Christmas disease). Hemophilia is discovered in the patient's childhood and with factor repletion the survival has increased greatly. Some patients take factor concentrates intravenously on a regular basis due to their low factor levels; however, some hemophiliacs only require factor replacement as needed. Hemarthrosis is the most common problem with both forms of hemophilia and, if treatment is withheld, can cause a severe, deforming arthritis. In cases of hemarthrosis, the effusion begins to be absorbed over the course of a week and will be gone in approximately 2 weeks. Occasionally, the hemophilia patient will present with life-threatening intracranial bleeds. More common are hematomas which can compress nerves, arteries, or veins causing a compartment syndrome. Retroperitoneal hemorrhage can also occur forming pseudo-tumors and compression of the femoral nerve.

7.2 History

A history of genetic diseases such as hemophilia, von Willebrand disease, or factor V deficiency should be discussed when dealing with an exquisitely tender joint. A history of anticoagulation and thrombocytopenia should also be discussed. A low-grade fever may be present with hemarthrosis but usually does not exceed 100.4 °F. A temperature higher than this could be a septic joint (see Chap. 2 on "Infectious Diseases"), although a septic joint is rare in hemophilia. In order from most common to least, the patient may report pain in the knees, ankles, elbows, shoulders, or hips. Occasionally, the small joints of the hands and feet are affected. A headache in a hemophiliac may be a life-threatening intracranial hemorrhage (ICH). Flank pain may be present with a retroperitoneal hemorrhage.

7.3 Exam

A low-grade fever not higher than 100.4 °F may be present with hemarthrosis. The joint in hemarthrosis will be tender and swollen and the patient will not want to move the affected appendage. A retroperitoneal hemorrhage may present with flank swelling (pseudotumor) and tenderness. An ICH may present with neurologic abnormalities (see Chap. 4 on "Neurology").

7.4 Diagnostics

An arthrocentesis may need to be performed to confirm hemarthrosis, usually in the ED. Drainage of the knee should not be undertaken. In unclear, less acute cases, a uric acid level, Lyme serology, and plain film of the joint(s) can be obtained fairly quickly.

Key Points
- Hemarthrosis in hemophilia requires ED referral to begin immediate infusion of factor VIII or factor IX.
- An exquisitely painful joint effusion without a clear diagnosis should be referred to the ED to rule out a septic joint.

8 Sickle Cell Disease

Sickle cell disease is caused by stiff, malformed red blood cells (RBCs) that damage the microvasculature.

8.1 General Considerations

Sickle cell disease is a prototypical genetic disease caused by a single amino acid substitution in the hemoglobin gene, glutamic acid to valine, in the B2 globulin component of hemoglobin. This mutated hemoglobulin causes a changed structure and behavior of the RBC such that the venules are damaged by the passage of the deformed RBC. This "sickled" RBC abnormally adheres to the endothelium causing ischemia in the microvasculature and veno-occlusion. Veno-occlusion or even frank infarction occurs in many systems including the lungs, central nervous system, liver, kidneys, bones, and joints. As such, the clinical symptoms of sickle cell disease are many, with pain crises in the musculoskeletal system being a major cause of morbidity and ED referral. Acute chest syndrome is another common outcome of sickle cell disease which can be life-threatening. Sickle cell disease is usually diagnosed in childhood, but milder phenotypes can be diagnosed in adulthood such as hemoglobin SC and sickle thalassemia.

8.2 History

Usually the diagnosis of sickle cell disease will be established in the patient. Extremes of temperature, vigorous exercise, anxiety, and infection are the usual precipitants of a pain crisis. The patients will often bypass the clinic to get treatment via a patient-controlled analgesia (PCA) pump in the hospital. Pain crises can occur anywhere on the body and can last anywhere from a few hours to 2 weeks. Some crises can be managed at home with aggressive oral hydration and oral analgesics. Sickle cell patients have an increased risk of osteomyelitis in unusual locations such as the spine due to *Salmonella*. Acute chest syndrome, a dreaded complication of sickle cell disease, is characterized by chest pain, shortness of breath, fever, and cough. Differentiating acute chest syndrome from other diagnoses such as pneumonia or pulmonary embolism is difficult.

8.3 Exam

Tender joints and diffuse pain are typical in pain crises. Fever, pulmonary crackles, and decreased oxygen saturation are common in acute chest syndrome.

8.4 Diagnostics

Sickle cell disease is characterized by a baseline hemolytic anemia and reticulocytosis. Hematuria is also frequently found in sickle cell patients.

Key Points
- Sickle cell disease is a systemic illness which affects a number of different organ symptoms with typical resultant symptoms.
- Pain crises and acute chest syndrome are common emergent complications of this disease.

Further Reading

Cydulka, R.K. Fitch, M.T., Joing, S.A., Wang, V.J., Cline, D.M., Ma OJ (Eds.) (2018) Tintinalli's emergency medicine manual (8) McGraw Hill, New York.

DeSouza S, Angelini D. Updated guidelines for immune thrombocytopenic purpura: expanded management options. Cleve Clin J Med. 2021;88(12):664–8.

Manzullo EF, Gonzalez CE, Escalante CP, Yeung SJ. Oncologic emergencies. New York: Springer; 2016.

Ophthalmology

Gregory M. Booth and Susan Tsu Thai

1 Introduction

1.1 General Considerations

True vision loss is always an emergency. Likewise, the red painful eye should always raise suspicion for an ophthalmic emergency. If there is ever a doubt, a same day ophthalmology consult is ideal; however, sometimes this is not easy to arrange. Furthermore, sometimes an immediate consult is not necessary, and the primary care clinician has time to give an initial treatment and follow the patient until ophthalmology consultation is available. Checking the patient's vision with the Snellen chart in the office is often useful. Normal vision is a valuable piece of information and should always be documented. Checking the vision, however, is often problematic as many conditions cause "blurry" vision that causes inability to accurately assess the visual acuity. In this case, the clinician has to rely on other elements of the evaluation to decide on the course of action. The chapter is divided into two parts. Painful vision loss/impairment will be covered first followed by painless vision loss.

G. M. Booth (✉) · S. T. Thai
Baltimore, MD, USA
e-mail: Boothg444@yahoo.com; Slt21122@yahoo.com

© The Author(s), under exclusive license to Springer Nature Switzerland AG 2022
G. M. Booth, S. Frattali (eds.), *Managing Emergencies in the Outpatient Setting*, https://doi.org/10.1007/978-3-031-15270-2_12

2 Painful Vision Loss

2.1 Chemical Exposure

2.1.1 General Considerations

Most chemical exposures of the eye will present to the ED and will bypass the office. However, the primary care clinician may occasionally have a patient who presents to the clinic initially by chance or by proximal location to the office.

The case is pretty straightforward as the patient needs emergent specialized care. While awaiting the ambulance or the ophthalmology appointment to be set up, initial treatment should be instituted. This consists of topical anesthetic drops such as proparacaine and irrigation of the eye. Sometimes up to 10–15 L, ideally of saline or lactated ringers, may be required. The irrigation should be continued until the pH is normal or for 30 min if pH strips are not available.

Key Point
- While setting up emergency care, IRRIGATE.

3 Major Trauma

3.1 General Considerations

Most significant trauma will bypass the office. However, some general principles apply.

3.2 Exam

Vision loss is possible depending on amount and type of trauma; however, lacrimation often makes this difficult to evaluate. Photosensitivity and conjunctival redness are common. Hyphema (blood in the anterior chamber see Fig. 1) or

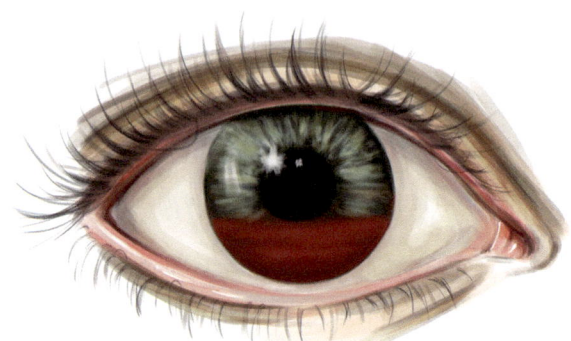

Fig. 1 Figure of hyphema caused by blood in the anterior chamber. Trauma may also lead to pupillary defects. Illustration by Olivia Welling

abnormally shaped pupil can be seen with trauma and requires immediate referral.

4 Minor Trauma

4.1 General Considerations

Minor trauma often causes abrasions in the epithelium of the cornea, the thick clear connective tissue that is anterior to the iris and pupil. *Corneal abrasions are not sight threatening* and do not require referral to an ophthalmologist unless the abrasion is very large or the patient wears contact lenses.

4.2 History

Corneal abrasions are very common in the primary care setting. Traumatic causes include tree branches, makeup brushes, and workplace debris. Workplace history is helpful in those who work with wood and metal. Sand is a common cause, especially with rubbing of the eye. Foreign body sensation is typical. The clinician should ask about contact lens use as this changes the approach.

4.3 Exam

The key to the exam is fluorescein staining and visualization with a cobalt blue light. The yellow dye will accumulate in the abrasion and fluoresce under the blue light. Simple corneal abrasions will show linear or geographic staining and usually do not require an ophthalmologist if small and uncomplicated. The eyelid should also be everted to look for fluorescing foreign bodies.

Special attention needs to be paid to eye pain in the case of the contact lens wearer. Contact lens use can cause a corneal abrasion that is not traumatic. The staining of a corneal abrasion from contact lenses is often different than that of a traumatic abrasion and will have punctate lesions that coalesce into a round defect (see Fig. 2). These lesions definitely require an ophthalmologist, and the size and symptoms determine if it is the same day or not.

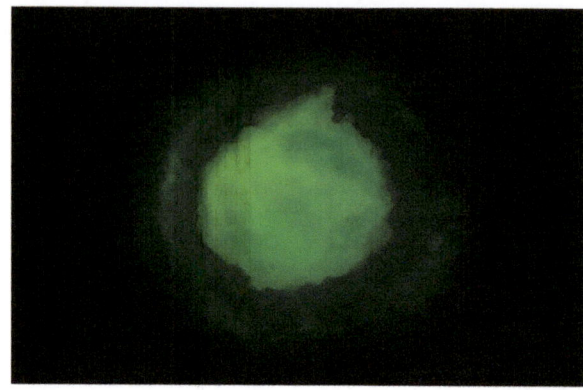

Fig. 2 Figure of corneal abrasion in a contact lens wearer. The circular defect will be apparent on fluorescein staining. Illustration by Olivia Welling

4.4 Treatment

Antibiotic eye drops which cover Pseudomonas in the case of the contact lens wearer. Patching is controversial but can decrease painful blinking and is often prescribed for 24 h.

Key Points
- Unless the patient is a contact lens wearer, corneal abrasion does not usually require specialist care.
- Corneal abrasion in a contact lens wearer requires anti-pseudomonal topical antibiotics and urgent referral (can wait until the next day or two if relatively small and uncomplicated and the pain is controlled).

5 Keratitis

Keratitis is characterized by an infiltrate of inflammatory cells into the cornea, the thick clear connective tissue that is anterior to the iris and pupil.

5.1 General Considerations

An estimated 930,000 outpatient office visits and 58,000 ED visits for keratitis or contact lens disorders occur annually. Keratitis can be spontaneous but is usually caused by infections or inflammatory diseases such as rheumatoid arthritis and ankylosing spondylitis. Keratitis should be seen by the ophthalmologist as soon as possible.

5.2 History

Keratitis is differentiated from a simple conjunctivitis by significant pain. Conjunctivitis usually causes burning and discharge. In contrast, the patient with keratitis will often be very photophobic and also have pain with accommodation. The pain is often severe and described as a deep ache.

5.3 Exam

A white spot or opacity can sometimes be seen over the cornea with ambient light. Fluorescein staining should be performed in all patients with significant eye pain and will accentuate the abnormality in keratitis. Herpes keratitis associated with herpes zoster (shingles) or herpes simplex demonstrates dendritic uptake on fluorescein staining (see Fig. 3) and also requires urgent referral. Zoster keratitis is predicted by zoster lesions at the tip of the nose called the Hutchinson's sign 90% of the time (see Fig. 4). However, this sensitive sign is not specific for keratitis or retinitis. Zoster lesions on the eyelid also necessitate urgent referral.

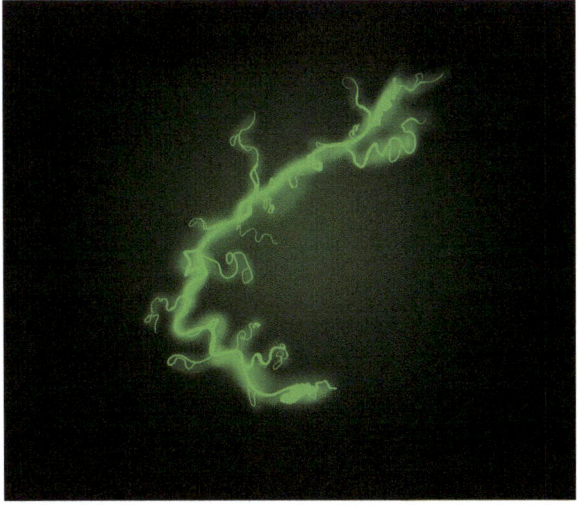

Fig. 3 A representation of herpes keratitis. Note the dendritic fluorescein uptake. Illustration by Olivia Welling

Fig. 4 Hutchinson's sign. Note the red papules on the nasal fold

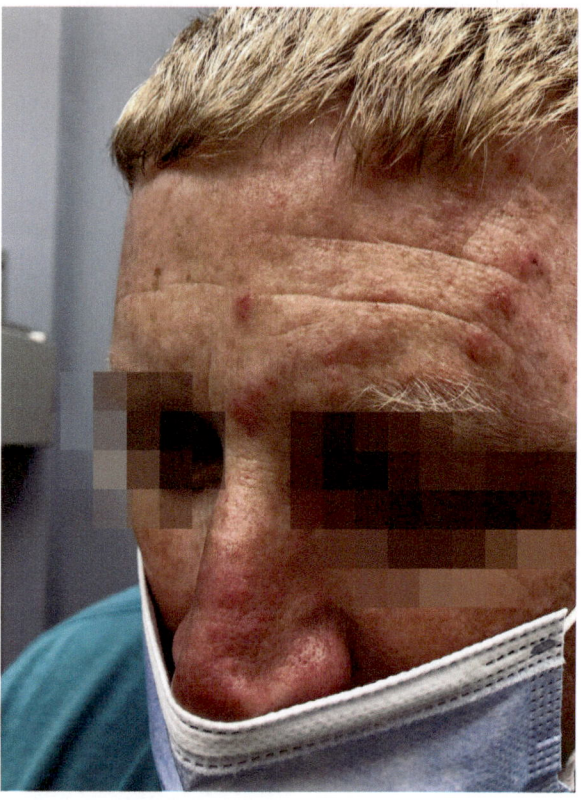

5.4 Treatment

As per the ophthalmologist. Antibiotics, antifungals, antivirals, etc. for infections and anti-inflammatories for inflammatory causes.

Key Points
- Keratitis is characterized by an infiltrate over the iris or pupil accentuated by fluorescein staining and needs immediate referral as does the dendritic lesion seen in herpetic keratitis.
- Hutchinson's sign is usually seen in herpes zoster keratitis.

6 Scleritis and Uveitis

Scleritis is inflammation of the thick white connective tissue of the globe. The uvea comprises the posterior compartment of the eye and uveitis can be categorized into anterior uveitis (iritis) and posterior uveitis (retinitis).

Ophthalmology

6.1 General Considerations

Approximately 400,000 cases of scleritis and uveitis occur in the U.S. each year. Like keratitis, the most common cause of scleritis and uveitis is infection or rheumatologic diseases (sometimes undiagnosed at time of presentation).

6.2 History

Like keratitis, scleritis and uveitis are characterized by significant pain. In contrast, conjunctivitis usually causes burning and discharge and will not cause severe pain unless very advanced. Scleritis will often have significant night pain. The patient with uveitis will often be very photophobic.

6.3 Exam

In scleritis and uveitis, extraocular eye movements may cause pain. The redness of the globe will be more central around the pupil in uveitis (see Fig. 5) as opposed to in the corners of the eyes as in conjunctivitis. In iritis, the pupil may be distorted, but reactive. There is often pain with accommodation and consensual pupillary reflex. The globe itself may be tender to the touch. Vision loss can occur and the vision should be checked using the Snellen chart.

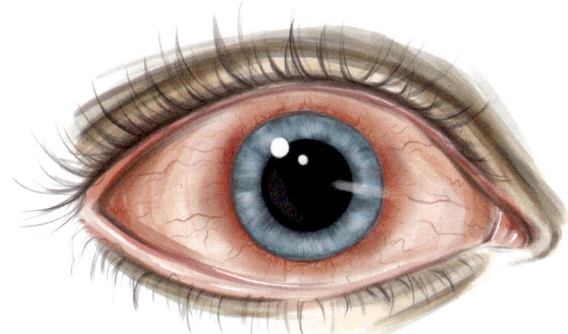

Fig. 5 Figure of anterior uveitis. Notice the inflammation around the iris referred to as ciliary flush. Illustration by Olivia Welling

6.4 Treatment

Like keratitis, treatment is per the ophthalmologist using antibiotics and anti-inflammatories. Surgery is sometimes necessary.

Key Points
- Significant pain often indicates inflammation of the deeper structures of the eye.
- Both scleritis and uveitis are emergencies and should be seen by a specialist as soon as possible.
- When the vision is intact and the symptoms and exam are of moderate severity, the patient may be able to wait until the next day.
- Topical antibiotics should be started and steroids should be avoided until seen by the ophthalmologist.

7 Endophthalmitis

Endophthalmitis is inflammation, most likely from bacterial infection, in the posterior of the visual structures of the eye (retina).

7.1 History

This most commonly occurs *post-procedure* and is characterized by rapidly progressive pain, red eye, discharge, and vision loss.

7.2 Exam

There is often a markedly inflamed eye and hypopyon (layered collection of white material in the anterior chamber of the eye) (Fig. 6) which are inflammatory cells.

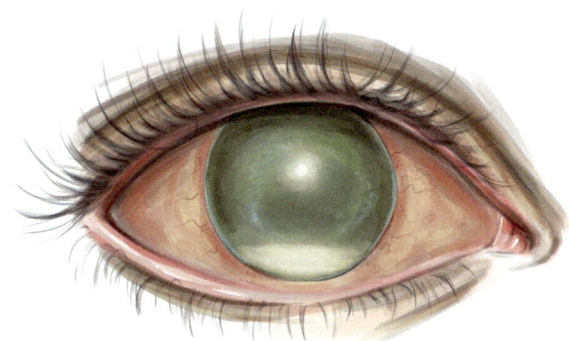

Fig. 6 Figure of endophthalmitis. Notice the layer of white cells (hypopyon) in the anterior chamber. Illustration by Olivia Welling

7.3 Treatment

Antibiotics and sometimes surgery.

Key Points
- Endophthalmitis will not be commonly seen in the clinic as the ophthalmologist will likely be called first.
- However, if the primary care provider gets called first or sees endophthalmitis in the clinic, it is an absolute emergency and requires immediate attention in the ophthalmologist's office (if possible) or the ED.

8 Optic Neuritis

Optic neuritis is characterized by inflammation and damage to the optic nerve leading to blindness.

8.1 History

Optic neuritis is relatively rare with approximately 25,000 cases occurring in the U.S. each year. Optic neuritis is commonly seen in young, adult, white patients. Traditionally, it is associated with multiple sclerosis; however, it is also seen with infectious etiologies, autoimmune disorders, and as an immune response to vaccination. The symptoms of optic neuritis are acute monocular vision loss, eye pain especially with movement, and reduced contrast to colors. Optic neuritis does not usually cause permanent vision loss.

8.2 Exam

The signs are vision loss (use Snellen chart) and afferent pupillary defect. The ophthalmologist will find optic disc edema in 1/3 of patients.

8.3 Treatment

The patient will need to be sent to a neuro-ophthalmology emergency department, likely for IV steroids.

Key Point
- A patient with sudden acute painful vision loss should be sent to an ED with neuro-ophthalmology expertise (if possible).

9 Acute Angle Closure Glaucoma

Acute glaucoma is characterized by increased pressure in the anterior chamber leading to severe symptoms and rapid vision loss if not treated quickly.

9.1 History

Risk factors are age over 50, female sex, and family history. Symptoms of acute glaucoma are severe nausea and vomiting, ocular pain, blurred vision, and headache. This can be difficult to distinguish from migraine as the symptoms are similar. They can be distinguished by the exam.

9.2 Exam

In acute glaucoma the clinician may find severe conjunctival injection, ciliary flush (see Fig. 5), corneal haziness, and a fixed dilated pupil. Vision loss is possible.

Key Points
- Acute glaucoma is characterized by a fixed dilated pupil on exam.
- Management of acute glaucoma is referral to an ED with ophthalmology expertise.

Ophthalmology 233

10 Orbital Cellulitis

Orbital cellulitis is a rare bacterial infection in the deep surrounding structures of the eye. It can lead to vision loss and spread of infection into the cranial cavity (i.e., meningitis).

10.1 General Considerations

With the extrapolation of data, approximately 3000 cases of orbital cellulitis occur each year in adults making this an extremely rare condition. Orbital cellulitis is much more common in children. Orbital cellulitis needs to be distinguished from the non-emergent condition of periorbital (or preseptal) cellulitis. Treatment for periorbital cellulitis is cephalosporins as this is a cellulitis. Augmentin or amoxicillin plus clindamycin are alternatives. Bactrim, if there is beta-lactam allergy, is an alternative. If there is high suspicion for orbital cellulitis, the patient should be referred to the ED for IV antibiotics. If concerning features are absent, then treatment for periorbital cellulitis can be started with short term follow-up.

10.2 History

Pain with extraocular eye movements can be present with both orbital and periorbital cellulitis though more prominent with orbital cellulitis. Double vision is a key symptom with orbital cellulitis. Decreased vision can be present in advanced cases though orbital cellulitis does not technically invade the globe itself.

10.3 Exam

If there is a significant fever, the patient most likely needs an emergent evaluation for orbital cellulitis. Both periorbital and orbital cellulitis have swelling and redness in the eyelids and the tissues surrounding the orbit and both may have conjunctival injection though such findings are more severe in orbital cellulitis. Orbital cellulitis also has signs of infection in the deeper structures of the orbital cavity such as proptosis, and cranial nerve palsies (reduction in extra ocular eye movements). Pupillary responses may be affected and afferent pupillary defect is an example.

10.4 Diagnostics

A CT scan of the orbits may help in the diagnosis.

Key Points
- Orbital Cellulitis requires IV antibiotics.
- Fever, if present, should be given strong consideration for referral to the ED.
- Other symptoms found will be that of periorbital cellulitis *plus* vision issues and/or signs of swelling behind the eye (proptosis and cranial nerve palsies).

11 Temporal Arteritis

Temporal arteritis also known as giant cell arteritis (GCA) is a systemic inflammatory disorder characterized by a variety of symptoms including headache and vision loss.

11.1 General Considerations

Temporal arteritis or giant cell arteritis (GCA) is not uncommon with 30,000 cases reported in the U.S. annually. GCA is a granulomatous vasculitis affecting various segments of the arterial tree. GCA is a disease of the adult population. The age of onset is generally older than 50 years of age with the average age being 70 years old. GCA is more common in women.

11.2 History

Headache is unilateral or bilateral and is located temporally in only 50% of patients and can be anywhere on the head. The headache can have an acute or subacute onset and is usually associated with other symptoms including jaw claudication which is specific but found only 30% of the time. The presence of polymyalgia rheumatica characterized by shoulder and sometimes hip pain without weakness of the muscles occurs in about 50% of patients with GCA. Systemic symptoms of fever, weight loss, and malaise are almost always present. One of the most alarming conditions is arteritic anterior ischemic optic neuropathy which is found approximately 15% of the time.

Ophthalmology

11.3 Exam

Signs include tenderness around the temples in the area of the temporal arteries. Sometimes, the temporal arteries are enlarged and inflamed, but this is not always the case. Vision loss is the most concerning exam finding, and the Snellen chart should be used to check for monocular vision loss. The typical findings are found on a dilated fundoscopic examination usually done by an ophthalmologist. An exam by an ophthalmologist can usually confirm the retinal findings associated with GCA.

11.4 Diagnostics

A complete blood count (CBC) should be checked for normocytic anemia. An erythrocyte sedimentation rate (ESR) rate >50 (a diagnostic criterion from the American College of Rheumatology) and elevated CRP are common. A normal CRP has a high negative predictive value. A temporal artery biopsy is often done later if the diagnosis is in doubt. The temporal artery biopsy can still be positive up to 2 weeks after the initiation of corticosteroids.

11.5 Treatment

If the patient is having vision loss, a referral to the ED for IV steroids is appropriate. If suspicion is high for GCA, but there is no vision loss, prednisone 60 mg a day should be started while awaiting laboratories and ophthalmology consultation. After diagnosis, patients are often referred to a rheumatologist as they require long term high dose steroids transitioning into a slow taper.

Key Points
- If the patient has a headache and vision loss, which is usually monocular (use Snellen chart), send to the ED for IV steroids.
- If the syndrome appears to be temporal arteritis without vision loss, the patient needs immediate prednisone 60 mg daily while attempting to confirm the diagnosis with immediate blood work, ESR and CRP.

12 Painless Vision Loss

12.1 Amaurosis Fugax and Central Retinal Artery Occlusion

These conditions cause painless vision loss and represent ocular strokes.

12.1.1 General Considerations

Reports of the incidence of amaurosis fugax vary but it is not uncommon. Amaurosis fugax and central retinal artery occlusion represent an ocular stroke and should be treated as such. Similarly, homonymous hemianopsia (see Chap. 4 "Neurology", Sect. 3) should also be treated as a stroke until proven otherwise. Risk factors for amaurosis fugax and central retinal artery occlusion are the typical stroke risk factors and include age (usually >50), smoking, diabetes, hyperlipidemia, hypertension, and obesity. Additionally, hyper-coagulable conditions (see Chap. 1 "Cardiovascular Disease") and autoimmune disorders have been associated with these entities. Estimation of the risk of large vessel stroke within 1–4 weeks of ocular stroke varies widely but is significant.

12.1.2 History

Amaurosis fugax is described as a shade descending down the whole field of vision from top to bottom, usually lasting 2–30 min. Amaurosis fugax is often intermittent. The symptom of central retinal artery occlusion is painless vision loss which can occur in seconds or develop over a matter of hours. Homonymous hemianopsia is loss of half of vision on the lateral sides of each eye and can be acute or subacute (see Chap. 4 "Neurology", Sect. 3).

12.2 Exam

Amaurosis fugax often can be seen on fundoscopic examination as a cholesterol plaque (called a Hollenhorst plaque) lodged within a retinal vessel (not always present). Central artery occlusion is the classic "cherry-red spot" at the macula on a gray membrane background on fundoscopic exam. It is caused by differential arterial supply to the retina. This may be difficult for the primary care provider to see. The exam for homonymous hemianopsia is evaluated by visual field confrontation with fingers held up in different quadrants to elicit the deficits (see Chap. 4 "Neurology", Fig. 1).

12.3 Diagnostics

These stroke syndromes require immediate carotid imaging. A CT angiography (CTA) of the head and neck or magnetic resonance angiography (MRA) are ideal.

12.4 Treatment

Aspirin 325 mg may be started in the case of amaurosis fugax.

Key Points
- Amaurosis fugax is described as a shade coming down over the eye and requires urgent imaging often in the ED depending on frequency.
- Sudden painless acute vision loss or the changes of homonymous hemianopsia in the absence of other visual symptoms represents a stroke until proven otherwise. The patient should be sent to the ED promptly.

13 Retinal Detachment

13.1 General Considerations

Retinal detachment is characterized by the peeling away of the retinal layer from the underlying pigment epithelium.

13.2 History

Risk factors include age, myopia (nearsightedness) diabetes, trauma, previous ocular surgery, and family history of retinal detachment. Symptoms are bright flashes peripherally in one eye then a shower of black dots or swarm of bees followed by loss of visual acuity. Alternatively, the patient will see brief recurrent flashes and floaters or a dark curtain or shadow moving from the outside in.

13.3 Exam

The primary care clinician makes the diagnosis historically and the patient may have abnormal vision.

13.4 Treatment

Immediate referral to retinal specialist for likely laser procedure to save vision.

Key Point
- Patients with visual symptoms of retinal attachment (see Sect. 13.2) need to see a retinal specialist immediately.

14 Pinguecula and Pterygium

Pinguecula (means fat in Latin) is a deposit of connective tissue on the conjunctiva of the eye. Pterygium (means wing in Greek—think pterodactyl) is a connective tissue deposit partially covering the iris. Neither causes vision loss and *neither one of these is an emergency*. Treatment: These two conditions do not need treatment unless they are symptomatic. Anti-inflammatory eye drops can be used if necessary. Ophthalmology for elective management if necessary or desired for pterygium.

Further Reading

Ameer MA, Peterfy RJ, Khazeani B. Temporal arteritis. Treasure Island, FL: Stat Pearls NIH; 2022.

Collier SA, Beach MJ, Yoder JS, Awsumb KL, Cope JR, MacGurn AK, Gronostaj MP. Estimated burden of keratitis—United States, 2010. Atlanta, GA: Centers for Disease Control and Prevention; 2014. Accessed 25 May 2022

Domingo E, Mashirfar M, Zabbo C. Corneal abrasion. Treasure Island, FL: NCBI Bookshelf. Stat Pearls NIH; 2020.

Freund PR, Chen SH. Herpes zoster ophthalmicus. CMAJ. 2018;190(21):E656. https://doi.org/10.1503/cmaj.180063.

Gu W, Tagg NT, Panchal NL, Brown-Bickerstaff CA, Nyman JM, Reynolds ME. Incidence of optic neuritis and the associated risk of multiple sclerosis for service members of U.S. Armed Forces. Mil Med. 2021. https://doi.org/10.1093/milmed/usab352.

Lagina A, Ramphul K. Scleritis. Treasure Island, FL: Stat Pearls NIH; 2022.

Murphy C, Livingstone I, Foot B, Murgatroyd H, MacEwen CJ. Orbital cellulitis in Scotland: current incidence, aetiology, management and outcomes: Table 1. Br J Ophthalmol. 2014;98(11):1575–8.

Riordan-Eva P, Augsburger JJ. Vaughan and Ashbury's general ophthalmology. 19th ed. New York: McGraw-Hill; 2017.

Shah SM, Khanna CL. Ophthalmic emergencies for the clinician. Mayo Clin Proc. 2020;95(5):1050–8.

Zhang Y, Amin S, Lung KI, Seabury S, Rao N, Toy BC. Incidence, prevalence, and risk factors of infectious uveitis and scleritis in the United States: a claims-based analysis. PLoS One. 2020;15(8):e0237995. https://doi.org/10.1371/journal.pone.0237995.

Dermatology

Gregory M. Booth

1 Introduction

Emergencies of the dermal, sub-dermal, mucosal, and submucosal surfaces are rare, but they will be encountered occasionally in the primary care setting. Stevens-Johnson Syndrome (SJS) and toxic epidermal necrolysis (TEN) are true emergencies requiring immediate hospitalization for supportive care. Pemphigus vulgaris is another true emergency requiring hospitalization for management. Vasculitis is a systemic disorder that requires hospitalization and has dermatologic findings that are characteristic of this entity. Angioedema is a sudden, potentially airway-threatening condition that requires monitoring in the emergency department.

2 Stevens-Johnson Syndrome (SJS) and Toxic Epidermal Necrolysis (TEN)

Stevens-Johnson Syndrome is a bullous desquamating rash affecting the skin and mucosal surfaces.

G. M. Booth (✉)
Baltimore, MD, USA
e-mail: Boothg444@yahoo.com

© The Author(s), under exclusive license to Springer Nature Switzerland AG 2022
G. M. Booth, S. Frattali (eds.), *Managing Emergencies in the Outpatient Setting*, https://doi.org/10.1007/978-3-031-15270-2_13

2.1 General Considerations

SJS affects all ages with highest incidence found in young adults between 20 and 40 years of age and occurs in males more than females. SJS is extremely rare with approximately 1300 cases occurring in the U.S. every year. The syndrome of SJS sits on a spectrum of disease that include toxic epidermal necrolysis (TEN). When less than 10% of the body surface area (BSA) is affected, SJS is considered the diagnosis. If the BSA affected is between 10% and 30%, the diagnosis is considered SJS-TEN overlap. When greater than 30% of the BSA is affected, TEN is considered the diagnosis. Patients with SJS are very vulnerable and should be hospitalized for supportive care. Like drug reaction with eosinophilia and systemic symptoms (DRESS) (see below), the cause is often identified to be medications especially lamotrigine (Lamictal) and sulfa drugs, but several infections such as HSV and mycoplasma pneumonia have also been identified as triggers and require treatment. Approximately half of the time, no etiology is unknown. The diagnosis needs to be established by biopsy as other bullous lesions such as paraneoplastic pemphigoid and pemphigus vulgaris (see Sect. 4) can masquerade as SJS. TEN is generally thought to be related to SJS and also affects all ages. TEN has a 25–35% mortality rate, although this has begun decreasing in recent years.

2.2 History

Fever, malaise, and myalgias may precede the condition. Pruritus may be present. Administration of a new medication 1–3 weeks prior is a common history. Like DRESS, anticonvulsants and antibiotics are often implicated. NSAIDs have also been cited as offending drugs. The lesions are described as painful or burning in the later stages.

2.3 Exam

The lesions are targetoid and may become bullous. Skin lesions begin as papules and macular lesions followed by the presence of target lesions 24–48 h later. Older bullous lesions may rupture or collapse with desquamation forming shallow ulcers. The mucosa is usually involved in two or more sites, such as the lips, oral mucosa, ocular mucosa, and anogenital mucosa. The pulmonary mucosa can be affected and cause a bronchitis or pneumonitis. Nikolsky sign (shearing of the skin with tangential manipulation) may be present in TEN as well as skin damage at sites of trauma. TEN is characterized by tender erythematous areas that become confluent within hours and develop into flaccid bullae and erosions with exfoliation.

2.4 Diagnostics

As mentioned, a biopsy is necessary (done in the hospital to confirm the case).

Key Points
- Stevens-Johnson syndrome is a potentially fatal condition affecting the skin and mucosal surfaces that need hospitalization for supportive care usually in a burn unit.
- Like DRESS (see below), the inciting factor is often medications, especially anticonvulsants and antibiotics.
- Toxic epidermal necrolysis is a rapidly progressive painful erythematous eruption that carries a high mortality.

3 Drug Eruption with Eosinophilia and Systemic Symptoms

Drug eruption with eosinophilia and systemic symptoms (DRESS) is a rash associated with the recent introduction of a medication.

3.1 General Considerations

Due to the shifting nomenclature and evolving classification of this drug eruption, exact information on incidence is difficult to ascertain, but severe cases of DRESS are known to be extremely rare. The pathogenesis of DRESS is unknown but is thought to be an immunologically mediated hypersensitivity syndrome. The organs affected by DRESS are primarily the liver followed by the brain, lungs, heart, and kidneys. The drug exposure defines the disease with DRESS typically occurring 2–6 weeks after initiation of the medication. Besides discontinuation of the drug, oral steroids in high doses are typical treatment options, sometimes needing to be prescribed for a month or longer. The mortality has been reported to be as high as 10% in untreated patients. Drugs that are commonly implicated in DRESS and SJS (see Sect. 1) are listed below, Anticonvulsants and antibiotics are the common culprits:

Allopurinol
Carbamazepine (Tegretol)
Lamotrigine (Lamictal)
Phenobarbital
Phenytoin (Dilantin)
Valproic acid (Depakote)
Minocycline
Piperacillin-tazobactam
Trimethoprim (Bactrim)
Sulfasalazine
Salazopyrin.

3.2 History

A rash forms 2–6 weeks after a drug is started. This rash may be pruritic but often there are no symptoms.

3.3 Exam

Early primary lesions are small 1–10 mm macules that coalesce into large patches of erythema (erythroderma). The lesions occur on the face, extremities, and trunk with a proclivity to the trunk. Edema can occur on the limbs and the face with facial swelling being a hallmark of the disease.

Lymphadenopathy may occur.

3.4 Diagnostics

The complete blood count will reveal eosinophils, sometimes in very high numbers. The effect on the liver is variable with the potential for fatal liver failure.

Key Points
- A diffuse rash associated with edema and eosinophilia and liver abnormalities on lab studies may represent the symptoms of the potentially fatal syndrome of DRESS.
- These patients must be monitored closely with a dermatologist, sometimes in an inpatient setting.

4 Pemphigus Vulgaris

Pemphigus vulgaris (PV) is a generalized, autoimmune, mucocutaneous, and blistering eruption that carries a grave prognosis.

4.1 General Considerations

The incidence of PV varies widely among different geographic locations and ethnicities but is estimated to be about 1–5 cases per million individuals. PV has a predilection for the Jewish and Hispanic heritage and typically affects older adults who are 40–60 years of age. The disease is characterized by bullous lesions and has a 90% mortality rate if untreated. Even when treated, PV still has a significant mortality rate of 10%. Treatment is oral steroids 40–60 mg daily followed by a slow taper. In severe cases, IV medications must be used to control the condition. A biopsy is necessary to make the diagnosis. On rare occasions, PV is drug induced with captopril and rifampin as common culprits and, rarely, beta-lactam antibiotics. Typically, the disease follows a chronic course; however, spontaneous remissions have been known to occur.

4.2 History

A history of recent medication initiation may be related as above. The lesions rupture and cause crusting and painful ulcers.

4.3 Exam

The lesions are flaccid vesicles and bullae that can reach up to several centimeters in size. Scaling and crusting of older lesions often lead to erosions. Mucosal involvement occurs 90% of the time and often in the oral mucosa, symptoms which can sometimes be confused with Stevens-Johnson Syndrome (SJS). The Nikolsky sign may be present (shearing of the skin with tangential pressure).

4.4 Diagnostics

A biopsy should be performed in the hospital to confirm the diagnosis.

Key Points
- Pemphigus Vulgaris (PV) is a severe vesiculobullous disease associated with cutaneous and usually mucosal involvement.
- Depending on the severity, patients may need to be admitted for IV steroid treatment.

5 Purpura and Vasculitis

Purpura can be the sign of a severe systemic illness.

5.1 General Considerations

Petechiae and purpura are caused by a variety of potentially fatal medical conditions. Various infections cause petechiae and purpura (see Table 1) Meningococcemia (see Chap. 4 "Neurology") and disseminated gonococcal vasculitis (see Chap. 2 "Infectious Disease", Sect. 4) and endocarditis (see Chap. 2 "Infectious Disease") are infections associated with petechiae and purpura that require hospitalization. Rocky Mountain spotted fever (RMSF, see chapter "Infectious Disease", Sect. 14) is another potentially fatal infectious disease characterized by petechiae and purpura.

The thrombotic microangiopathic anemias (HUS and TTP) can cause petechiae and purpura (see Chap. 5 "Nephrology"). Immune thrombocytopenic purpura (ITP) also causes petechiae and purpura (see Chap. 11 "Hematology"). Vasculitis in the form of Henoch-Schonlein purpura (HSP) and cryoglobulinemia are systemic illnesses that require prompt attention to avoid potential morbidity and mortality. HSP is typically a disorder of children 2–10 years of age but can affect any age. Bowel infarction and hemorrhage may occur with HSP as can renal failure. However, HSP is often self-limited and is associated with permanent sequelae <10% of the time. Cryoglobulinemia is an immunogenic disorder associated with infections (hepatitis B and C), collagen vascular diseases, and hematologic cancers. The pathophysiology of cryoglobulinemia is delineated into three types. Type I is associated with hematologic cancers. Type II is caused by all three types of associated diseases. Type III is limited mainly to infection (Hep C) and collagen vascular diseases. Cryoglobulin disease is generally a disease of the adult and geriatric population and the treatment is management of the underlying illness. Other entities of less clinical consequence can cause palpable purpura in isolation such as leukocytoclastic vasculitis (LCV), or hypersensitivity vasculitis, seen as an allergic reaction to medications. The collagen vascular diseases such as lupus can also cause LCV of varying severity (see Table 1).

Table 1 Common causes of petechiae and purpura (not an exhaustive list). The disorders of immune thrombocytopenic purpura (ITP), thrombotic thrombocytopenic purpura (TTP), and hemolytic uremic syndrome (HUS) also cause petechiae and purpura. Anti-neutrophil cytoplasmic antibody (ANCA) vasculitides may also have petechiae and purpura

Infections	Vasculitis
Endocarditis	Cryoglobulinemia
Disseminated gonococcal infection (DGI)	Henoch-Schonlein purpura (HSP)
Meningococcus	Leukocytoclastic Vasculitis (collagen vascular disease and hypersensitivity)
Rocky mountain spotted fever (RMSF)	ANCA vasculitides

5.2 History

Fever, headache, and non-blanching petechiae could be meningococcus or rocky mountain spotted fever (RMSF). The presence of a tick bite or the systemic symptoms seen with RMSF may differentiate these entities. A swollen painful joint in a young sexually active patient is consistent with DGI. HSP is a systemic illness often causing headache, arthralgias and arthritis, and gastrointestinal symptoms. An upper respiratory infection often precedes HSP. However, pharyngitis from group A streptococcus (GAS) and various bacterial and viral illnesses can also precipitate this IgA-mediated vasculitis. Cryoglobulinemia is a systemic vasculitis often characterized by arthralgias, myalgias, and abdominal pain in older adults. Neurologic (wrist or foot drop) and pulmonary symptoms may also be present with cryoglobulinemia.

5.3 Exam

Palpable purpura is a raised, non-blanching, purple papule usually on the lower extremity. The rash of disseminated gonococcus is few in number and are small isolated papules with surrounding erythema. These papules may coalesce into ecchymosis (see Fig. 1) or ulcerate. Various findings may also be associated with petechiae and purpura depending on the clinical scenario such as murmur with endocarditis, neck stiffness or rigidity with meningococcus, or a swollen joint with DGI. A wrist drop or foot drop may be present with cryoglobulinemia.

5.4 Diagnostics

A complete blood count (CBC) should be obtained to assess for hematologic malignancy and severe thrombocytopenia. Renal failure is commonly seen with vasculitis and will be evident by a rising creatinine and an active sediment on urinalysis (protein, red cells, and red cell casts—see chapter "Nephrology" for full details). LFTs should be drawn to assess liver function. An evaluation for palpable purpura without a diagnosis includes complement levels, RF, ANA, HIV, hepatitis B and C, and cryoglobulins (if inpatient). A chest radiograph or CT may be informative in some situations. If an infectious source of vasculitis is suspected, throat cultures for GAS, urine studies for chlamydia and gonococcus, and blood cultures are appropriate.

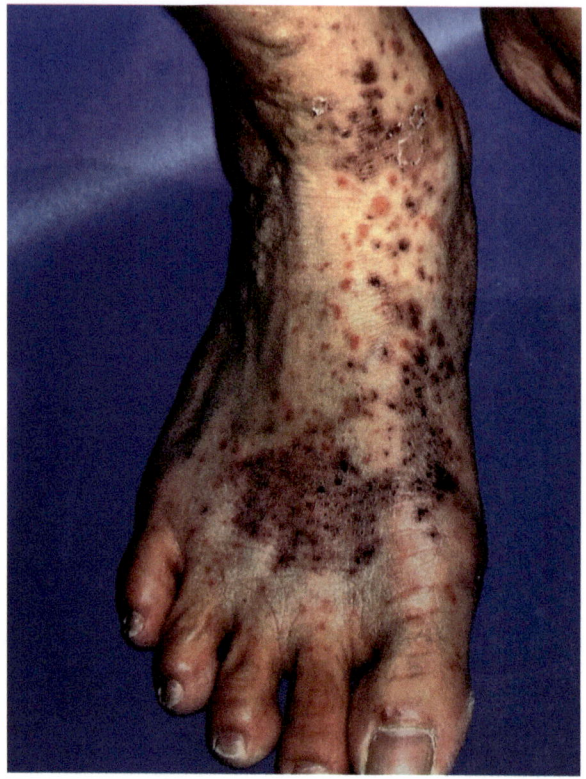

Fig. 1 Petechiae and purpura in the lower extremity of a patient with Henoch Shonlein purpura (HSP). Used with permission from Fitzpatrick, J.E., High, W.A. (2018) *Urgent care dermatology: symptom-based diagnosis.* Elsevier

Key Points
- Palpable purpura is associated with a variety of illnesses that require prompt attention and care, often in a monitored setting.
- Petechiae and purpura without associated symptoms can be due to medications and are benign. These benign conditions should have normal labs.

6 Angioedema

Angioedema is the non-pitting edema of subcutaneous and submucosal surfaces.

6.1 General Considerations

Angioedema can affect the lips, oral cavity, neck, extremities, gut, and becomes life-threatening if the larynx is involved. Severe episodes of angioedema associated with respiratory distress must be monitored in the ED where there is easy access to tracheostomy equipment. Angioedema may be classified according to three mechanisms: (1) histaminergic (allergens and medications), (2) bradykinin-mediated [ace inhibitors, angiotensin receptor blockers (ARBs) and C1 deficiency], and (3) prostaglandin pathway associated (NSAIDs). Almost any drug or allergen can be associated with histaminergic angioedema. The histaminergic form is treated with antihistamines, corticosteroids, and in severe cases, epinephrine. Bradykinin-mediated forms (i.e., ace inhibitors, ARBs, and C1 deficiency) are more resistant to treatment. C1 deficiency may be either hereditary (hereditary angioedema) or acquired and is not associated with urticaria. The hereditary form generally has a more severe presentation, is associated with abdominal symptoms, and is the major cause of fatal angioedema. Hereditary angioedema presents in childhood and young adulthood. Approximately, 80% of patients with hereditary angioedema have a relative with angioedema. Hereditary angioedema is on the differential for generalized edema. Acquired C1 esterase inhibitor deficiency is another cause of C1-mediated angioedema and can be associated with neoplasms, infections, and medications. The treatment for attacks of C1-mediated angioedema is plasma derived C1 esterase concentrate. Icatibant, a bradykinin-receptor antagonist, is another on-demand treatment for hereditary angioedema.

6.2 History

A history of medications should be elicited. Patients may report pruritus and rash as well as swelling in the throat and mouth. Allergen induced angioedema generally develops within an hour of exposure and lasts 1–2 days. Ace inhibitor or ARB angioedema may occur any time but is most common within the first week of starting the medication. Attacks in hereditary angioedema generally take a day to develop and last 2–3 days. Swelling of the bowel wall can cause abdominal pain which is most often seen in hereditary forms of angioedema.

6.3 Exam

Swelling of the lips and surrounding tissues with or without urticaria is the defining characteristic of angioedema. Wheezing and rhonchi may be heard on lung exam. Usually, patients with C1 mediated angioedema (hereditary angioedema) do not have associated urticaria which clinically differentiates hereditary from histaminergic angioedema due to allergens and medications. Patients with hereditary angioedema can have a serpentine, erythematous, non-pruritic rash.

6.4 Diagnostics

A low serum C4 is a sensitive but non-specific test to define angioedema. Mast cell tryptase levels are usually normal in hereditary but not in acquired angioedema.

If a low C4 is detected, a quantitative and functional C1-INH test should be drawn to further evaluate the angioedema.

Key Points
- Severe attacks of angioedema associated symptoms and signs of respiratory compromise need to be monitored in the ED.
- A C4, tryptase level, and C1-INH testing may be drawn to assess for the diagnosis.

7 Viral Infections in the Immunosuppressed

Severe viral infections of the skin and mucosa can occur in immunosuppressed patients.

7.1 General Considerations

On rare occasions, severe viral infections of the herpes family can occur in immunosuppressed patients (HIV patients, transplant patients, and those on corticosteroids). Severe herpes simplex virus (HSV) 1 and 2 infections can occur in the oral, genital, and anal mucosa which require intravenous IV acyclovir. HSV meningoencephalitis (see Chap. 4 on "Neurology") and HSV keratitis (see Chap. 12 "Ophthalmology") also require an emergent response with intravenous (IV) acyclovir. Severe varicella zoster virus (VZV) infections can occur in a dermatomal fashion or disseminate and also require IV acyclovir.

7.2 History

Burning lesions in the anogenital mucosa may be present in HSV infections. Rashes may be present either in a dermatomal distribution or be more widely disseminated in VZV infection. Neurologic manifestations may be present in HSV and VZV encephalitis. Visual symptoms may be present with HSV keratitis or VZV keratitis and retinitis.

Dermatology

7.3 Exam

HSV and VZV rashes are characterized by a vesicular eruption that can develop into erosive lesions. HSV and VZV may cause CNS infections and a full neurologic exam should be done.

7.4 Diagnosis

Polymerase chain reaction (PCR) tests on vesicular fluid can be performed in unclear cases. HIV tests should be performed in unusual or severe HSV or VZV cases.

Key Points
- Severe HSV or VZV skin infections can require IV acyclovir.
- Neurologic or visual manifestations may accompany the skin eruption.

Further Reading

Fitzpatrick JE, High WA. Urgent care dermatology: symptom-based diagnosis. Amsterdam: Elsevier; 2018.

Ingold CJ, Khan MA. Pemphigus vulgaris. Treasure Island, FL: NIH Stat Pearls; 2021.

Memon RJ, Vivekanand T. Angioedema. Treasure Island, FL: NIH Stat Pearls; 2021.

Walsh SA, Creamer D. Drug reaction with eosinophilia and systemic symptoms (DRESS). Clin Exp Derm. 2010;36:6–11.

Yang M, Lee JY. Incidence of Stevens-Johnson syndrome and toxic epidermal necrolysis: a nationwide population-based study using national health insurance database in Korea. PLoS One. 2016;11(11):e0165933.

Psychiatry

Gregory M. Booth

1 Introduction

Mental health compromises a major part of any primary care practice. A large proportion of symptoms and problems presenting in a primary care practice are related to underlying psychiatric disorders. Therefore, primary care physicians should be acutely aware that the cause of many physical symptoms originate from mental stress and psychiatric disorders. Most patients who have depression and anxiety are treated in the primary care setting; hence, primary care physicians must be able to perform a basic psychiatric mental status exam and generate an appropriate diagnosis. Basic psychopharmacology should also be emphasized in order to treat these patients.

2 Depression and Anxiety

Depression and anxiety are two of the most common mental health issues encountered in primary care. While they may seem obvious, symptoms will differ in degree of severity and distress for the patient. The physician must be vigilant while questioning patients, as sometimes it is not easily evident that the patient has depression and anxiety. Anxiety can cause chest pain, shortness of breath, headaches, and muscle tension. Common symptoms of depression are sadness, fatigue, poor

---

G. M. Booth (✉)
Baltimore, MD, USA
e-mail: Boothg444@yahoo.com

© The Author(s), under exclusive license to Springer Nature Switzerland AG 2022
G. M. Booth, S. Frattali (eds.), *Managing Emergencies in the Outpatient Setting*, https://doi.org/10.1007/978-3-031-15270-2_14

concentration, low motivation, and vague pain or exacerbation of pain syndromes. While not life-threatening, these symptoms can build up over time and lead to serious morbidity and mortality, with suicide being the ultimate outcome in some situations. Suicide should be constantly considered in any patient presenting with depression.

3 Suicide

3.1 General Considerations

According to The American Foundation for the Prevention of Suicide, 132 suicides occur every day, and men are 3.5 times more likely to commit suicide. Suicide is a devastating but preventable outcome, so every effort should be made in the outpatient setting to help those at risk. As such, screening tools for depression are often part of the triage process in ambulatory clinics. Suicidal ideation (SI) is a broad term that is often used and will be discussed further under history and physical exam. Risk factors for SI can be viewed as static (in the past) or dynamic (current stressors). The most important static factor is past suicide attempts and a family history of suicide. Other static issues are a history of severe depression, substance abuse, and physical/mental abuse. A dynamic risk factor is access to lethal means such as firearms or a cache of medications. Other dynamic factors are social stressors, such as finances (loss of job), social issues (divorce or break up), or recent homelessness. Severe social stressors are associated with the most risk, especially when occurring suddenly. Intoxication is also a dynamic risk factor, and intoxicated, unstable individuals must be sent to the ED. Psychosis is another dynamic risk factor contributing to instability as discussed below.

3.2 History

When a patient complains of a depression affecting their life functions, the provider should ask questions to define the depths of the depression. A good introductory question to this topic is "are you preoccupied with thoughts of death"? "Have you had thoughts of self-harm? " is a more specific question and should also be asked. If the patient admits to suicidal ideation, further questions can be asked such as: "Are the thoughts vague? Do you have a plan? Do you plan on acting soon?" Part of the calculus is protective factors, which can be extrinsic (strong social relationships, feeling that others rely on them), or intrinsic (good coping skills, strong belief systems). A patient's religion can be ambivalent since some religions believe that suicide is the ultimate sin while others believe their God will forgive them.

3.3 Exam

The physical exam in psychiatry is standardized; but, in the context of suicidality should focus on clues to the stability of the patient. A disheveled appearance or poor hygiene should be noted. Speech patterns can be described regarding volume (speaking too softly) and rate (too slow or too fast). The activity of the patient should be noted: are they agitated, or do they show psychomotor retardation? While the mood is the reported expression of feelings, the affect is the outward appearance of mood. The physician should ask themselves: does the patient appear sad, angry, etc.? Is the affect congruent? For example, does the patient appear sad when discussing a death and happy when discussing the birth of a child? These attributes can indicate if the patient is organized and in control or could possibly commit a rash act.

3.4 Diagnostics

None unless the patient has altered mental status (see below).

Key Points
- Evaluation for the safety of ambulatory patients is complex as delineated above.
- If the overall gestalt of the patient is low risk, make sure they have outlets for emergency support. The national suicide prevention hotline is one such resource (800-273-8255).

4 Psychosis

Psychosis is generally defined to be loss of contact with reality, a disorder of thought.

4.1 General Considerations

It is estimated that between 0.25% and 0.5% of people in the USA suffer from a psychotic disorder. One hundred thousand teenagers and adults in the USA have an initial psychotic event each year. New-onset psychosis is generally considered an unstable medical condition because the patient is a danger to themselves and others. Possible causes of psychosis are psychiatric illnesses such as mood and thought disorders, drug intoxications, drug withdrawal, or medical illness. A red flag for a medical cause of the psychosis is a patient older than 45 with no psychiatric history. While it is somewhat unusual to see cases of psychosis in the outpatient primary care practice, it is important to be aware of such cases when they present. Patients that present with psychotic symptoms require a special set of skills that are not within the primary care purview.

4.2 History

The history is critical to diagnosing psychosis. The key to diagnosing psychosis is defining the various disorders of thought that are present. Disorganization is evidenced by tangentiality, a non-linear thinking pattern lacking a consistent theme. Conversely, perseveration may be present as evidenced by intense focus on one line of thought and difficulty moving on to a new topic. Delusions are more organized and elaborate, consisting of fixed, false beliefs that predominate a patient's thinking. Hallucinations affect the senses, producing false auditory, visual, tactile, or other sensory perceptions. More subtle findings may be present such as editing, which are pauses in speech to avoid expression of odd ideas or experiences.

4.3 Exam

The exam is closely related to the history. The patient's general appearance and hygiene are often affected. The patient may be observed responding to internal stimuli, such as moving their head to visual stimuli, or talking to themselves in response to auditory stimuli. The patient may be obviously agitated or aggressive due to dysphoria from the psychotic condition.

4.4 Diagnostics

In new-onset psychosis (in the absence of a previous diagnosis of a psychiatric disorder), a full laboratory evaluation is necessary to rule out secondary causes of psychosis, typically done in the ED. A full workup for psychosis includes a drug screen and some of the tests listed under altered mental status and delirium (see Sect. 5.4).

Key Point
- Patients found to have a profound, new-onset disorder of thought need expedited care in the ED to rule out a serious medical disorder and often to protect themselves and others.

5 Altered Mental Status and Delirium

5.1 General Considerations

Altered mental status is considered an acute disruption of brain function in several domains including cognition, orientation, motor, and sensory functions. Many medical causes of altered mental status (and by extension - delirium) have been covered in this manual. One of the most common causes of altered mental status is medication (anticholinergics, benzodiazepines, and opiates). Other causes are interruptions of the CNS by infections, hypoxia, hypercarbia, endocrine disorders, disorders of sodium homeostasis, malignant hypertension, withdrawal, toxins, vitamin deficiencies, etc. Delirium is a related syndrome also characterized by acute brain dysfunction that waxes and wanes over time and can be considered a more insidious form of altered mental status. Though delirium is frequently a syndrome found in the inpatient setting, it may occasionally be encountered in the outpatient setting. This is a serious consideration, given that there are numerous underlying medical conditions that can lead to delirium. It can be even more difficult when patients are elderly, have preexisting medical conditions, dementia, and/or psychiatric conditions. Dementia is a permanent, gradual decrease in brain function occurring over time, and is a risk factor for delirium. It can be difficult to differentiate from delirium and both can occur at the same time. Those 65 and older are at greater risk for delirium. Whereas altered mental status nearly always calls for an immediate higher level of care, the subacute course of delirium can sometimes allow for a more deliberate evaluation. However, very often patients need to be sent to the hospital for a proper medical workup. Considering the complexity of these conditions, the patient's history and exam must be reviewed carefully.

5.2 History

A detailed personal, psychiatric, and family history can be revealing, with the chronicity of the symptoms being an initial focus. Much of the history will be given by family and friends and may be confusing. Delirium can be hypo or hyperactive. The patient may be withdrawn intermittently and display muscular findings consistent with retarded catatonia such as muscle weakness while conscious. Hyperactive delirium is often associated with agitation, heightened arousal, and hypervigilance. Mood changes can be reported as can hallucinations and delusions.

5.3 Exam

Vitals should be normal, including pulse oximetry. The physical exam should also be normal. A full mental status examination is unnecessary to identify a patient with a high risk for delirium. The patient may be disoriented; inattention and an altered level of consciousness may also be observed. Memory impairment and disorganized thinking may be exhibited as can perceptual disturbances. The patient may exhibit psychomotor retardation or agitation. None of these findings are specific for any particular etiology of delirium, and they are present in other psychiatric presentations and medical causes of altered mental status. Ascertaining the cause of the alteration in brain function must be based on the clinical scenario.

5.4 Diagnostics

A urinalysis can be obtained in the office to evaluate for a urinary tract infection (a very common etiology for altered mental status in the elderly, usually not an emergency). A complete blood count may reveal findings consistent with an infection. A complete metabolic panel can reveal disturbances in glucose and electrolytes as well as renal and hepatic dysfunction. A thyroid stimulating hormone (TSH), vitamin B12, and RPR (syphilis) are very common laboratories to order in scenarios of subacute altered mental status.

Key Points
- Acute altered mental status usually requires immediate evaluation.
- Subacute, fluctuating altered mental status (delirium) in some circumstances may be investigated as an outpatient.

6 Withdrawal Syndromes

6.1 General Considerations

Various legal and illegal substances can cause lethal syndromes when abruptly withdrawn. Alcohol, benzodiazepines, and barbiturates can cause lethal withdrawal while amphetamines, cocaine, marijuana, and opiates cause debilitating but not life-threatening symptoms. It is common for patients with substance abuse issues to request opioids and other addictive medications in a primary care setting. To complicate things, the primary care clinician is often not aware of the patient's underlying addiction problems. At this time, most states give clinicians online access to a patient's opioid prescription history which helps to manage those who may abuse legal narcotics. The most common life-threatening withdrawal syndrome is alcohol related withdrawal syndrome (AWS) and will be encountered in clinical practice at the primary care level. In a very broad sense, alcohol use disorder (AUD) is common with a prevalence around 14% and lifetime incidence of 29%. Over half of patients who drink heavily do not experience withdrawal symptoms at all, while some will experience delirium, seizures, and death. Typically, at least 2 weeks of heavy drinking is necessary to create a withdrawal scenario. Once alcohol abuse syndrome is identified, abrupt cessation and history of withdrawal symptoms should be assessed. These symptoms occur due to the unopposed response to the cessation of the pharmacologic depressive effects of alcohol on the nervous system. AWS severity can be quantified to aid in disposition with the CIWA-Ar or SAWS scoring symptoms. Considering AWS presents with varying severity, patients seeking medication (benzodiazepines) to treat withdrawal symptoms represent a treatment dilemma. One issue is the prescription of a potentially lethal number of sedatives to a psychiatrically unstable patient. Social situations such as caregiver support, transportation, and housing are other considerations. Another issue is the lack of durable treatment for alcoholism often encountered with such a prescription for outpatient management.

6.2 History

Patients frequently present with a history of chronic alcohol use. A history of prior withdrawal is important to elicit. A consumption of greater than eight drinks per day is a risk factor for complicated withdrawal. Two weeks of heavy drinking followed by reduction or cessation of alcohol is usually required to produce symptoms of withdrawal. The symptoms usually begin within a 6–48-h period and include anxiety, nausea, confusion, memory impairment, restlessness, headache, and insomnia. The patient may report sensory disturbances such as sensitivity to light, sound, or sensation of pins and needles or burning on the skin. The patient may also report seeing or hearing things that they know are not there.

6.3 Exam

Vitals may be abnormal indicating autonomic hyperreactivity with blood pressures and pulse elevated above normal levels. Sweating may be observed or felt upon examination. Agitation may be observed, varying from mild restlessness to pacing. A mild tremor may be felt fingertip to fingertip, or moderate when observed with arms extended. A severe tremor can be observed at rest without arms extended. The presence of moderate to severe tremor indicates a more severe withdrawal course. Tactile, auditory, and visual disturbances can be present and be of varying severity. Observation of itching or excessive attention to the skin is a sign of withdrawal. The patient may be easily frightened or have frank auditory hallucinations. The examiner may observe sensitivity to light or frank visual hallucinations. These disturbances indicate the possibility of a more severe course of withdrawal. Safe transportation should be the most pressing concern for visibly intoxicated patients.

6.4 Diagnostics

A CBC, CMP, urine drug screen, and blood alcohol level are labs commonly obtained in relation to a withdrawal syndrome. A blood alcohol level, if present, does not correspond to a patient's level of intoxication. Significant abnormalities upon laboratory investigation provide additional support for a monitored setting for management of alcohol withdrawal.

Key Points
- Alcohol withdrawal should be managed in a controlled setting if possible.
- The CIWA-Ar and SAWS scales can quantitate the degree of withdrawal and aid in deciding disposition.
- The presence of a significant tremor is a sign that a moderate withdrawal syndrome will be encountered.
- Abnormal labs indicate the possible need for a monitored setting.

7 Neuroleptic Malignant Syndrome (NMS)

Neuroleptic malignant syndrome (NMS) is a constellation of symptoms and signs caused by dopamine receptor blockade in the CNS.

7.1 General Considerations

Neuroleptic malignant syndrome (NMS) is extremely rare but is very serious when it does occur. Care should be taken to not miss this diagnosis as mortality is considerable (5–20%). NMS is an idiosyncratic reaction caused by dopaminergic blockade in the CNS. As an idiosyncratic reaction, NMS may occur at any time and does not require any change in medication dosage. Unlike serotonin syndrome (see below), the onset can be gradual. The typical antipsychotics (1st generation) are most commonly associated with this syndrome; however, any medication that blocks dopamine may cause this syndrome. Therefore, atypical antipsychotics can cause NMS. Other medications such as prochlorperazine (Compazine) and promethazine (Phenergan) have also been implicated. Abrupt changes in dopamine within the CNS can also promote NMS as seen in drug holidays for Parkinson's patients. The constellation of symptoms is the tetrad of hyperthermia, autonomic dysfunction, rigidity, and altered mental status (AMS). In practice, NMS presents on a spectrum and not all four elements are necessary for the diagnosis. The diagnosis is clinical and requires the exclusion of other diagnoses. Malignant catatonia is a related condition that causes hyperthermia, autonomic instability (without hypertension), and delirium, but is associated with various characteristic movements unlike the rigidity found in NMS. Malignant catatonia is also an emergency; the treatment is electroconvulsive therapy. NMS is not to be confused with malignant hyperthermia which causes a similar syndrome in response to certain medications used in anesthesia.

7.2 History

The history of a dopamine modulating drug (antipsychotic) is the key to the diagnosis, and any patient on these drugs should be considered for NMS when a fever is encountered with the vital signs. AMS is the hallmark finding and may be reported as confusion or more profound disturbances of sensorium.

7.3 Exam

Fever greater than 100.4 °F or 38 °C will be present. Autonomic instability is manifested by HR >100, tachypnea, and diaphoresis. An elevated blood pressure distinguishes this from an infectious etiology. The pupils will be dilated. Reflexes will be increased and a tremor may be present. Rigidity is a hallmark of NMS.

7.4 Diagnostics

A CPK will be found to be >4 times normal. The CSF will usually be normal.

Key Points
- Dopamine antagonist exposure or dopamine agonist withdrawal in the presence of a fever greater than 100.4 °F on at least two occasions should raise suspicion for NMS.
- Treatment is supportive with liberal use of benzodiazepines after hospitalization.

8 Serotonin Syndrome (SS)

Serotonin syndrome (SS) is a constellation of symptoms and signs due to increased serotonergic activity in the CNS.

8.1 General Considerations

The true incidence of serotonin syndrome is unknown due to under-diagnosis of mild cases, but fatal cases are relatively rare. Serotonin syndrome (SS) is an overreactivity of the serotoninergic system in the CNS due to a medication overdose or drug-drug interaction, (different from the idiosyncratic reaction of neuroleptic malignant syndrome). Unlike neuroleptic malignant syndrome (NMS), the onset is more rapid, occurring over the course of hours. SSRIs are the most common medication involved in SS, either at high doses, overdoses, or in combination with other serotonergic medications. Other common serotonergic medications that may precipitate SS are:

- MAOIs (selegiline and phenelzine) (MAOIs cause the most severe and long-lasting cases.)
- Cyclobenzaprine

- Tramadol
- Illegal drugs such as Cocaine, ecstasy (MDMA), and amphetamines
- Tricyclics (amitriptyline and nortriptyline)
- Anti-seizure drugs (valproate and carbamazepine)
- Herbals (St. John's Wort)
- Linezolid (antibiotic).

The clinical picture is very similar to NMS, with the physical finding of clonus being a differentiating feature. Treatment of SS is similar to NMS with supportive care and liberal use of benzodiazepines in the hospital setting. Cyproheptadine, an early antihistamine, has anti-serotonergic activity and has also been used as treatment, especially in refractory cases. The recovery is usually rapid.

8.2 History

The usual finding is some type of modification or overdose of serotonergic medications. Altered mental status is typical. Restlessness is present. GI upset including nausea, vomiting, and diarrhea may be present and helps differentiate this from neuroleptic malignant syndrome (NMS).

8.3 Exam

A fever and autonomic instability (elevated blood pressure, heart and breathing rates with diaphoresis) are likely present. Tremor and muscle rigidity may also be present. Hyperreflexia is also common. The pupils will be dilated. These symptoms are also found with NMS, but the defining feature of SS is clonus. Clonus can be elicited by a forced dorsiflexion of the foot which is followed by involuntary "beats" of plantar flexion.

8.4 Diagnostics

Like NMS, the diagnosis is clinical and no investigation is pathognomonic.

Key Points
- A change in the level of serotonergic activity in the CNS by initiation of a medication, increase in dosage, or drug overdose can cause serotonin syndrome (SS).
- The syndrome can cause hyperthermia, autonomic instability, and rigidity.
- SS is clinically differentiated from NMS (see above) by the presence of clonus.

Further Reading

Nordstrom KD, Wilson MP, editors. Quick guide to psychiatric emergencies. New York: Springer; 2018.
Simon LV, Keenaghan M. Serotonin syndrome. Treasure Island, FL: NIH Stat Pearls; 2022.
Tiglao SM, et al. Alcohol withdrawal syndrome: outpatient management. Am Fam Phys. 2021;104(3):253–70.

Index

A
ABCD2 score, 100
Abdominal aortic aneurysm (AAA), 23
Abdominal pain, 71, 76, 154, 161, 203, 206
Abnormal uterine bleeding (AUB), 158
Acute glaucoma, 232
Acute kidney injury, 124, 126
　pre renal, 123, 124, 127, 128
　intrinsic, 123, 124, 128–130
　　glomerulonephritis, 128–130
　post renal, 123, 124, 131
Acute limb ischemia, 27
Acute liver failure, 88, 89
Acute myeloid leukemia (AML), 213
Acute rhinosinusitis (ARS), 181, 182
Acute suppurative thyroiditis, 208, 209
Adrenal crisis, 202, 203
Alcohol use disorder (AUD), 256
Allopurinol, 241
Altered mental status (AMS), 254–256, 258
Amaurosis fugax, 236
Anemia, 215, 216
Angioedema, 246, 247
Anticholinergics, 141, 142, 186
Antinuclear antibody (ANA), 188
Anti-Parkinson's drugs, 142
Anti-psychotics, 142
Anxiety, 251
Aortic dissection, 25, 26
Appendicitis, 78, 79
Arrhythmias, 9
Ascending cholangitis, 86, 87

Asthma, 185
Atrial fibrillation (AF), 10
Atrial flutter, 12
Atrioventricular nodal re-entrant tachycardia (AVNRT), 13

B
Bariatric surgery, 95
Bell's palsy, 109
Benign paroxysmal positional vertigo (BPPV), 177
Bitemporal hemianopsia, 104, 106
Bladder procedures, 141
Blood urea nitrogen (BUN), 125
Botulism, 120, 121
Bradyarrhythmias, 15

C
Cauda equina syndrome, 150, 151
Cerebrovascular accident (CVA), 100, 102–106
CHADS2-VASC score, 10–12
Chemical exposure, 224
Chikungunya, 62, 63
Cholecystitis, 80
Chronic liver disease, 89–91
Chronic myelogenous leukemia (CML), 213
Chronic obstructive pulmonary disease (COPD), 10, 185, 186
Clostridium botulinum, 120
Complete blood count (CBC), 61, 235

Congestive heart failure (CHF), 190
    diagnostics, 8
    dyspnea, 7
    edema, 7
    etiology, 7
    paroxysmal nocturnal dyspnea, 8
    tachycardia, 8
Constipation, 142
Coronary artery disease, 1–3
    chest pain, 2
    HEART score, 2
    myocardial infarction, 1
    Wellens syndrome, 4
CRB-65 rule, 46
Cryptogenic organizing pneumonia (COP), 188

D
Deep vein thrombosis (DVT), 18, 19, 132
Dengue, 60, 61
Depression, 251
Diabetic ketoacidosis, 195, 196
Diffuse alveolar hemorrhage (DAH), 189
Diphtheria, 70
Disseminated gonorrheal infection (DGI), 38
Diverticulitis, 81
Drug eruption, 241
Duke's criteria, 44

E
Ectopic pregnancy, 153, 154
Encephalitis, 110, 111
Endometriosis, 154
Endophthalmitis, 230
Endoscopic retrograde cholangiopancreatography (ECRP), 96
Enteric fever, 59, 60
Epiglottitis, 173, 174
Epistaxis, 165–168

F
Febrile travelers, 54
Foreign bodies, 183
Fournier's gangrene, 144, 145

G
Gastric volvulus, 85
Gastrointestinal bleeding, 93, 94
Giant cell arteritis (GCA), 234

Group A streptococcal (GAS), 29
Guillain-Barre syndrome (GBS), 117, 118

H
HEART score, 2
Hemarthrosis, 219
Hemolytic uremic syndrome (HUS), 129
Hemoptysis, 188, 189
Hernias, 85
Human immunodeficiency virus (HIV), 48, 49
Hypercalcemia, 136, 205, 206
Hyperemesis gravidarum (HG), 162, 163
Hyperglycemic hyperosmolar state (HHS), 197, 198
Hyperkalemia, 135
Hypermagnesemia, 137
Hypernatremia, 134
Hypertensive emergency, 28, 29
Hypertrophic cardiomyopathy (HOCM), 22
Hyperviscosity syndrome (HVS), 214, 215
Hypocalcemia, 136, 207, 208
Hypoglycemia, 198, 199
Hypokalemia, 134
Hypomagnesemia, 137
Hyponatremia, 133
Hypophosphatemia, 138

I
Infective endocarditis (IE), 43–45
Infertility, 154
Inflammatory bowel disease, 95
Interstitial lung disease, 187, 188
Intestinal volvulus, 85
Intrauterine device (IUD), 154, 157
Intrinsic renal disease, 128
Irritable bowel syndrome (IBS), 76

J
Jones criteria, 30

K
Keratitis, 226, 227

L
Legionella pneumonia, 66
Lemierre's syndrome, 172, 173
Leptospirosis, 57–59
Leukemia, 213

Index

M
Malaria, 55, 56
Malignant otitis externa, 176, 177
Mastoiditis, 174, 175
Measles, 66, 69
Meniere's disease, 178
Meningitis, 110
Mesenteric ischemia, 84
Microangiopathic hemolytic anemia (MAHA), 128
Minocycline, 241
Minor trauma, 225
Multifocal atrial tachycardia (MAT), 13
Multiple sclerosis (MS), 113, 114
Myasthenia gravis, 114, 115
Mycobacterium tuberculosis, 47
Myocardial infarction, 1
Myxedema, 201, 202

N
Nephrolithiasis, 139, 140
Neuroleptic malignant syndrome (NMS), 258, 260
Neurological conditions, 142
Neutropenic fever, 53
Non-steroidal anti-inflammatories (NSAIDs), 76, 82

O
Optic neuritis, 231
Orbital cellulitis, 233
Organ prolapse, 141
Orientia tsutsugamushi, 65
Osteomyelitis, 39, 40
Ovarian torsion, 155, 156

P
Pancreatitis, 91, 92
Paroxysmal nocturnal dyspnea, 8
Pelvic inflammatory disease (PID), 156–158
Pelvic schistosomiasis, 154
Pelvic tuberculosis, 154
Pelvic tumors, 141
Pemphigus vulgaris (PV), 242, 243
Penile fracture, 149
PERC score, 10, 16
Percutaneous endoscopic gastrostomy (PEG), 96
Pericarditis, 5, 6
Peripheral vascular disease (PVD), 39
Peritonsillar abscess (PTA), 168–170
Phenobarbital, 241
Pinguecula, 238
Pituitary apoplexy, 204, 205
Pleural effusion, 190, 191
Pneumonia, 45, 46
Pneumothorax, 192
Post-renal acute kidney injury, 131
Pre-eclampsia, 161, 162
Pre-renal acute kidney injury, 127, 128
Priapism, 148, 149
Prior abdominal surgery, 154
Prior ectopic pregnancy, 154
Prior infection (PID), 154
Prostatic hypertrophy, 141
Prostatitis, 143
Psychosis, 253, 254
Pulmonary embolism (PE), 15–17, 189
Purpura, 243
Pyelonephritis, 42

R
Renal vein thrombosis, 132
Retropharyngeal abscess, 170, 171
Rheumatic fever, 29–31
Rheumatoid factor (RF), 188
Rocky Mountain Spotted Fever (RMSF), 64, 65, 245

S
Salazopyrin, 241
Scleritis, 228–230
Seizure, 116
Sepsis
    diagnostics, 35
    hypotension, 33
    organ dysfunction, 33
    severe inflammatory response syndrome, 34
Septic arthritis, 38, 39
Serotonin syndrome (SS), 259, 260
Severe inflammatory response syndrome (SIRS), 34
Sexual assault, 163
Sickle cell disease, 220, 221
Sinus tachycardia (ST), 9
Small bowel obstruction (SBO), 82, 83
Soft tissue infections, 35–37
Spinal cord compression, 111, 112, 211, 212
Steven-Johnson Syndrome, 239, 240
Sudden sensorineural hearing loss, 179, 180

Suicide, 252, 253
Sulfasalazine, 241
Surgical site infections, 71
Syncope, 19, 20, 22
Systemic inflammatory response syndrome (SIRS), 34

T
Tachyarrhythmias, 9
Temporal arteritis, 234, 235
Testicular torsion, 145, 146
Thoracic aortic aneurysm (TAA), 24, 25
Thrombocytopenia, 217, 218
Thrombotic thrombocytopenic purpura (TTP), 129, 217, 244
Thyroid storm, 199, 200
Toxic shock, 34, 35
Transient ischemic attack (TIA), 100–102
Transplant patients, 51, 52
Transverse myelitis, 118
Traumatic brain injury (TBI), 107, 108
Tubal sterilization, 154
Tuberculosis, 47, 48

U
Unstable angina, 2
Urethral stone, 142
Urethral stricture, 142

Urinary retention, 141, 142
Urinary tract infection, 142

V
Vaginal bleeding, 158–161
Valproic acid, 241
Varicella zoster virus (VZV), 119, 248, 249
Vasculitis, 244, 245
Ventricular arrhythmias (VT), 14
Vertebral osteomyelitis, 41
Vertigo, 101, 103, 108, 114, 165, 175–180
Viral hemorrhagic fever, 66

W
Wellens syndrome, 4
Wells score
    PE, 10, 15, 16
    DVT, 18
Wernicke's encephalopathy, 119
Withdrawal syndromes, 256, 257
Wolff-Parkinson White syndrome (WPW), 14

Y
Yellow fever, 56, 57

Z
Zika virus, 63, 64

GPSR Compliance

The European Union's (EU) General Product Safety Regulation (GPSR) is a set of rules that requires consumer products to be safe and our obligations to ensure this.

If you have any concerns about our products, you can contact us on ProductSafety@springernature.com

In case Publisher is established outside the EU, the EU authorized representative is:

Springer Nature Customer Service Center GmbH
Europaplatz 3
69115 Heidelberg, Germany

Batch number: 08823208

Printed by Printforce, the Netherlands